the birthing cycle

what a woman needs to know about her pregnancy

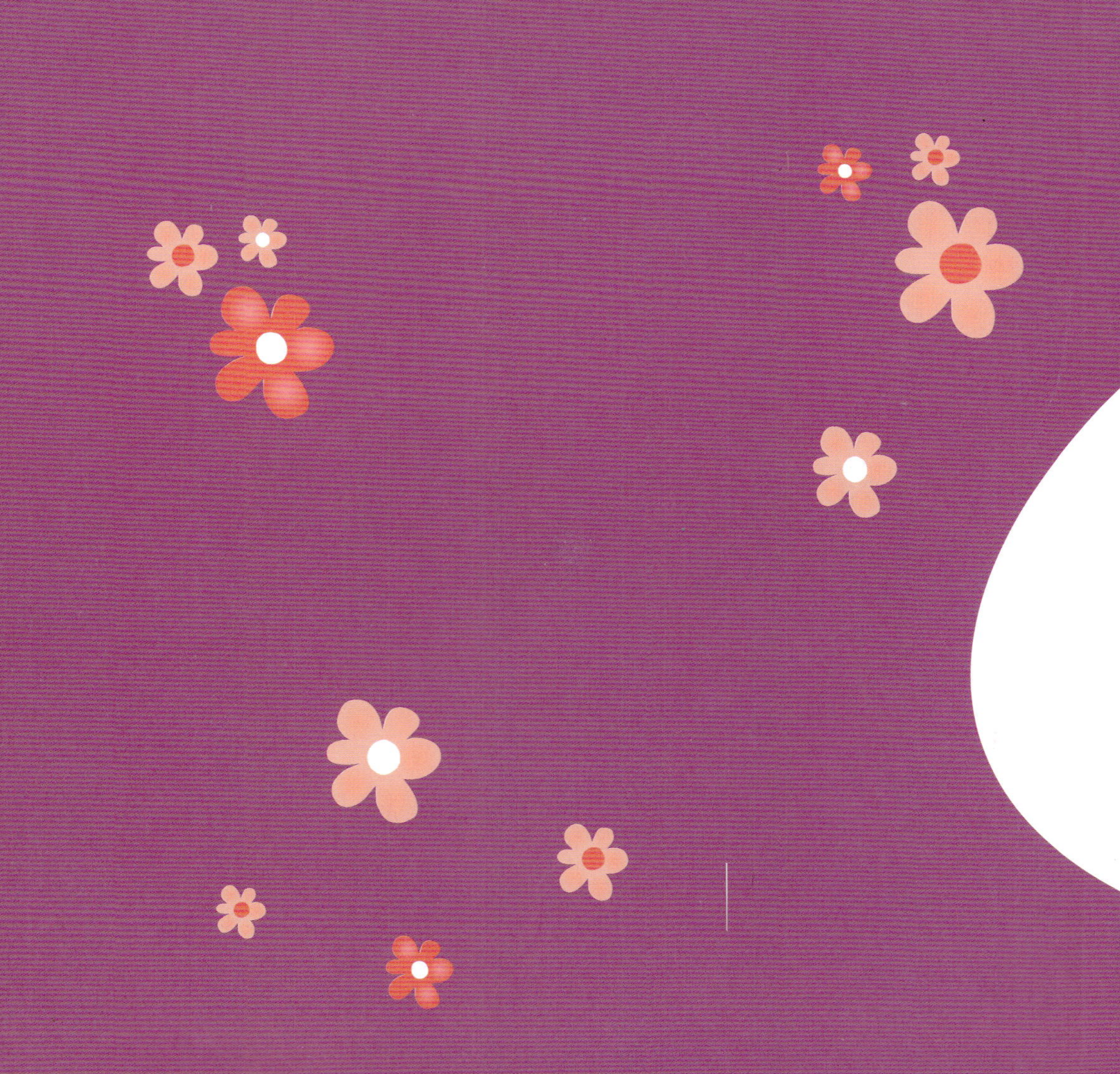

the birthing cycle
what a woman needs to know about her pregnancy

RONNIE SELLERS PRODUCTIONS
PORTLAND, MAINE

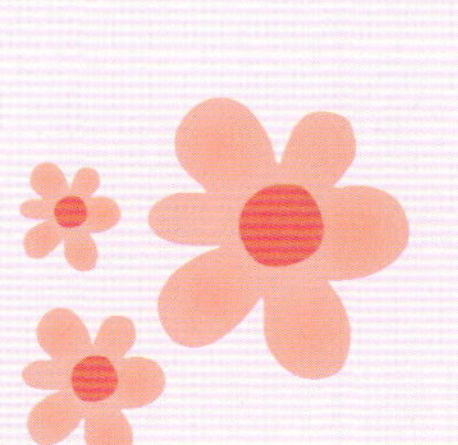

contents

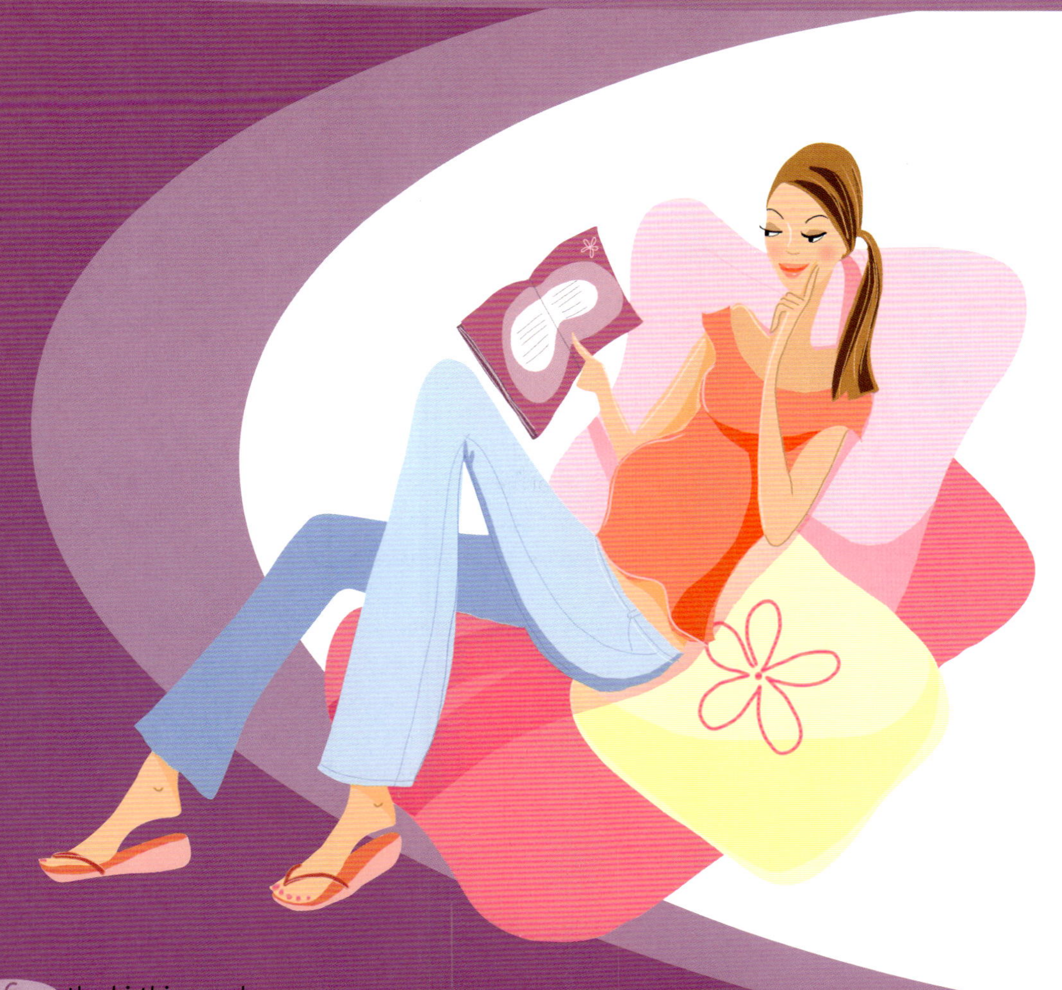
weeks
1 2 3 4 5 6 7 8 9 10 11 12 13 14 15 16 17 18 19 20 21 22

how to use this book

In just nine months, a minute single cell will become a small, but complete, person. At the same time, your body will adjust physically to provide your growing baby with all it needs to survive within your womb.

Although an entirely natural process, being pregnant can present challenges. In addition to significant physical changes, you'll experience a multitude of emotions ranging from anticipation and excitement to doubt and vulnerability. If the more negative feelings become applicable to you, don't panic. Many pregnant women (and their partners) experience similar emotions. You can minimize your anxieties simply by learning what to expect during each stage.

Following a brief introduction to the biological process of conception, this book offers a week-by-week guide to your baby's development and explains the physical and emotional challenges you are likely to face. In addition to a wealth of invaluable advice, you will also find journal pages where you can record your questions for your healthcare providers, and your personal thoughts and feelings as your pregnancy advances. While you are pregnant, this book will serve as a valuable guide to what's happening. Once your baby arrives, it will provide a record of this special time.

1 getting pregnant

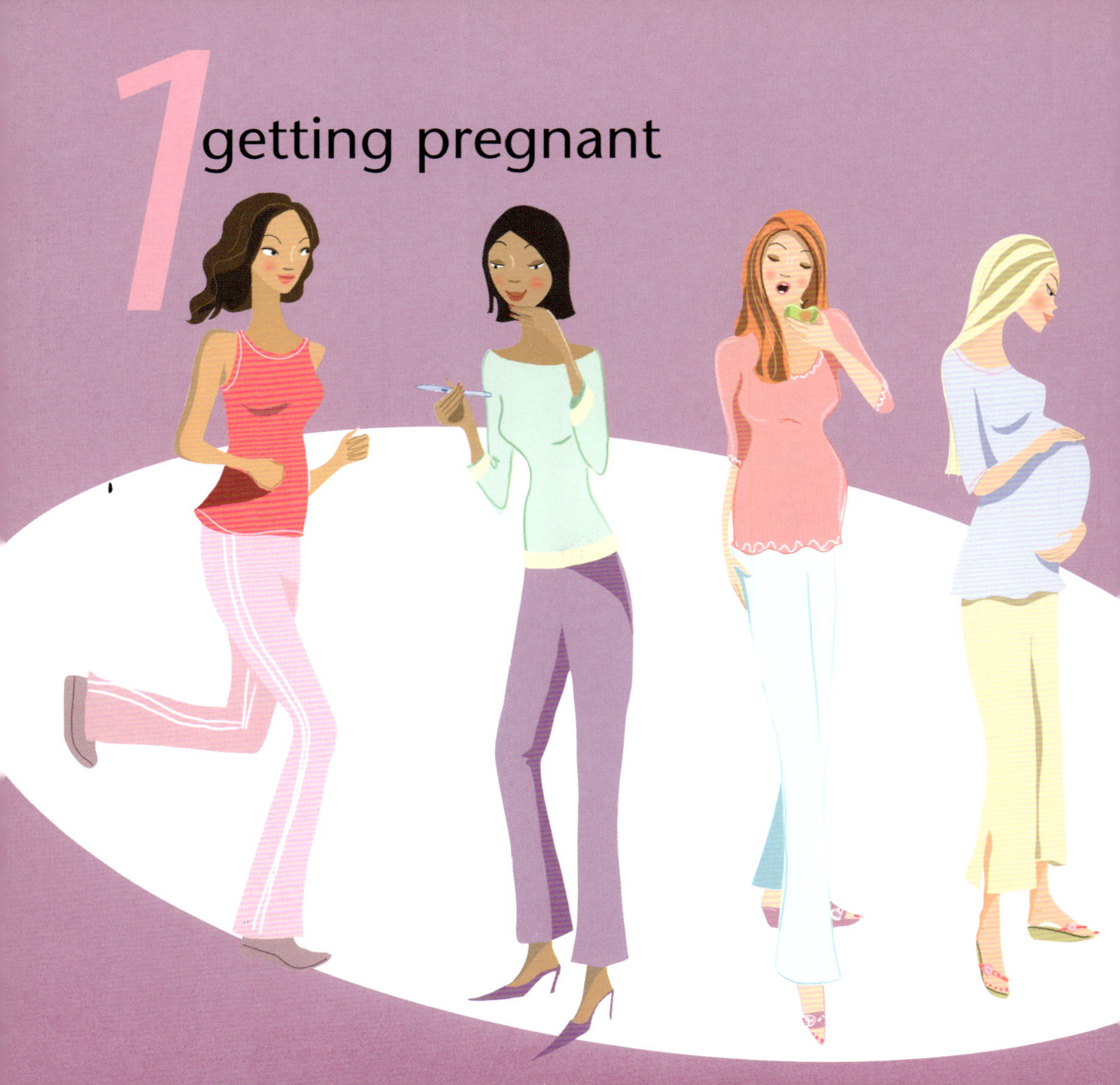

You've decided you want to have a baby. Soon you will try to conceive. But do you really know how it all works? This section of the book offers a useful refresher on your anatomy and the reproductive cycle, and describes how conception actually takes place. Here's your chance to prime yourself for the various physical changes you'll experience as soon as you become pregnant, and to find out what you can do to promote a healthy outcome right from the start.

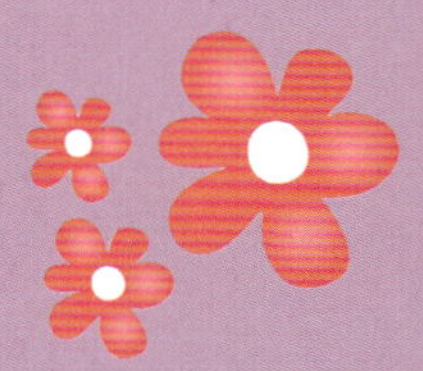

anatomically speaking

In order to be able to communicate effectively with your doctor and other caregivers during your pregnancy, it helps to be familiar with the key parts of your anatomy. It is also useful to know something about the chemistry behind the changes you are going to experience along the way.

know your body

Vagina: this is a tube connecting your uterus, or womb, to the outside world. Sperm pass through it into the uterus, and the baby passes out through it during birth. The vagina's internal surface is covered with ridges that allow it to stretch to accommodate the head of the baby.

Labia: raised folds of skin, often compared to lips, at the entrance to the vagina, or birth canal.

Perineum: a triangular-shaped mass of muscles and elastic fibers located between the vagina and anus. It's designed to stretch during childbirth.

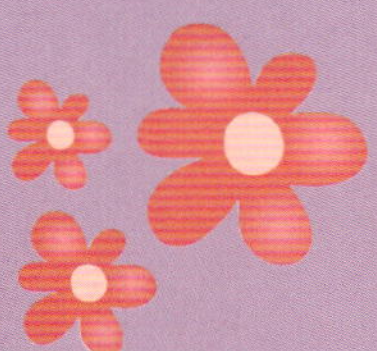

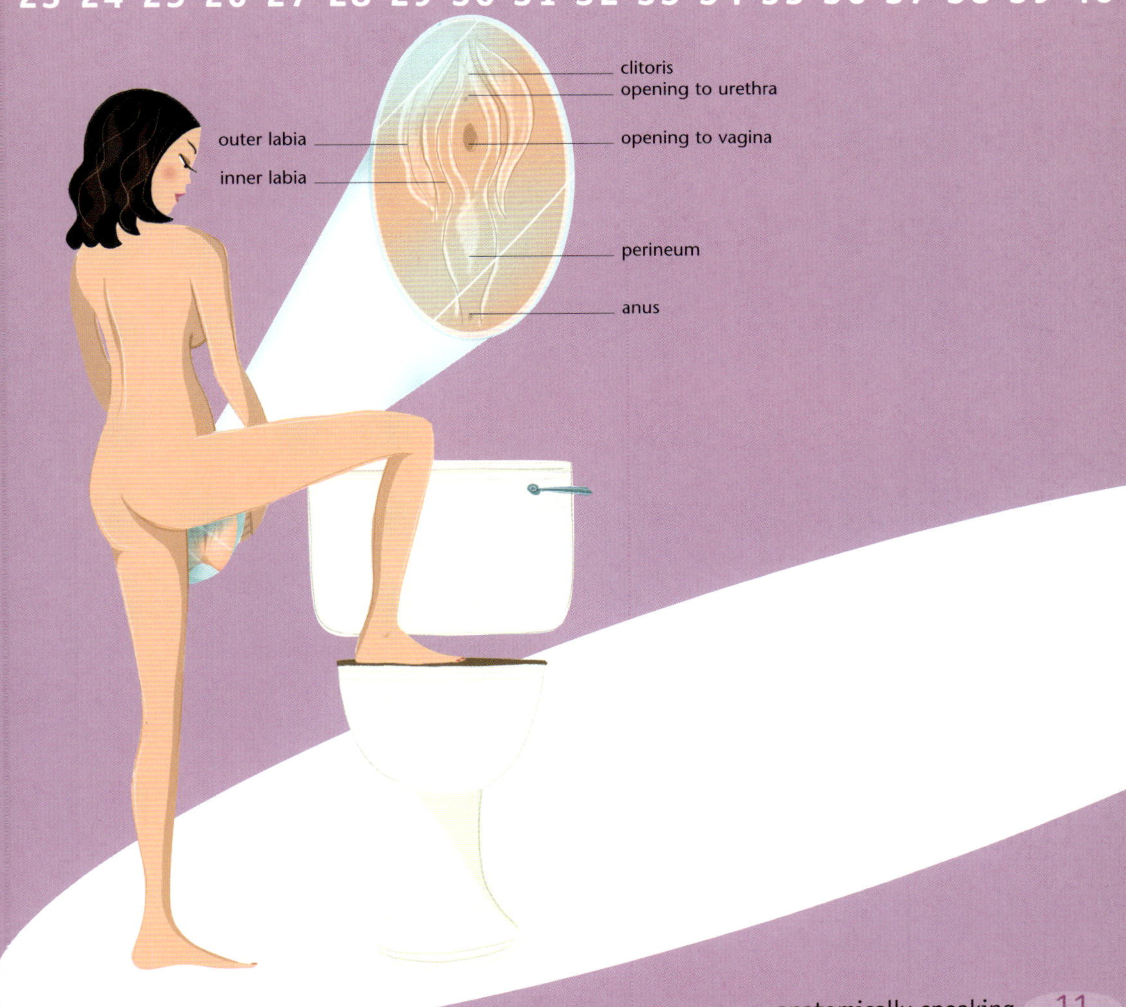
clitoris
opening to urethra
outer labia
opening to vagina
inner labia
perineum
anus

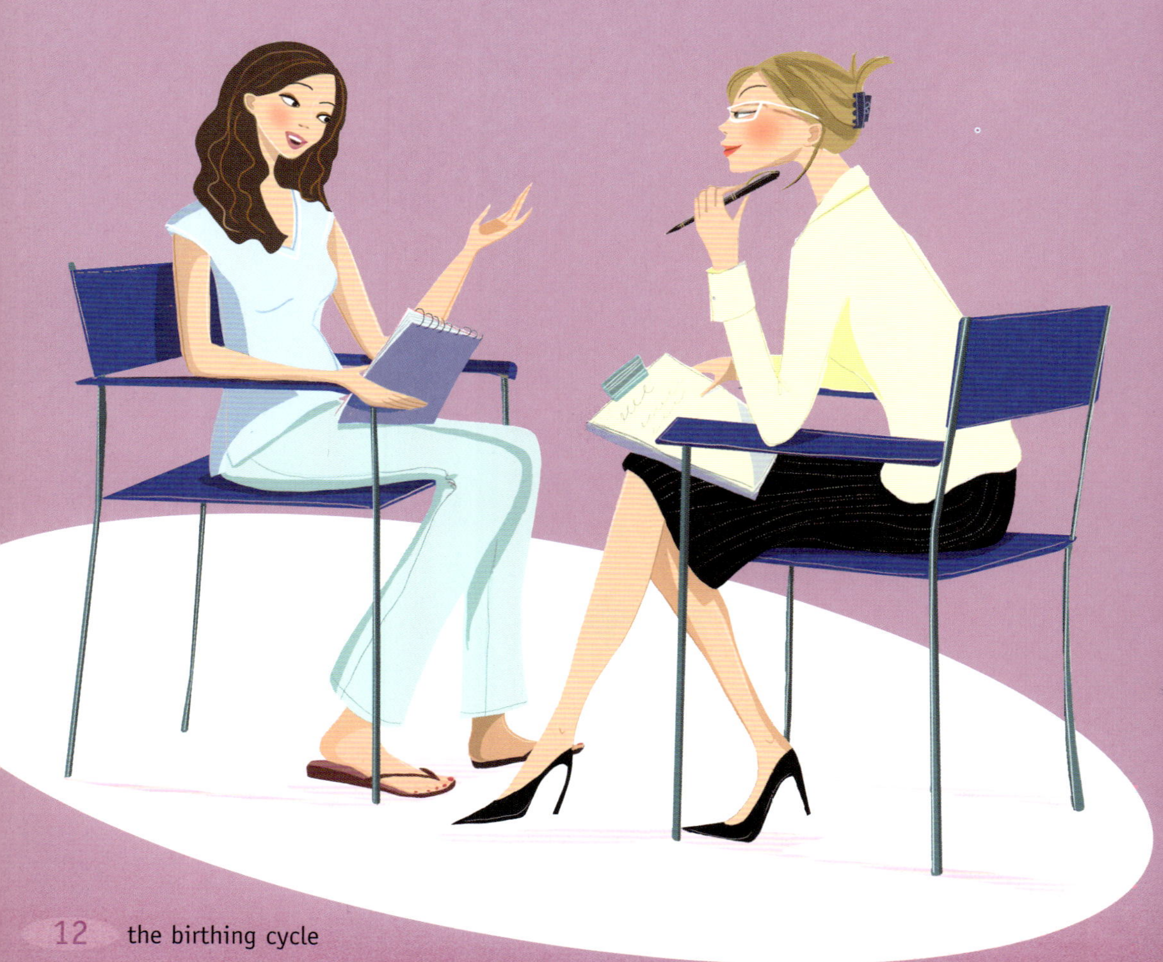

anatomically speaking

Located deep within your pelvis, your uterus, ovaries, and fallopian tubes play key roles in conception and in sustaining a pregnancy.

Cervix: this neck-shaped opening at the top of the vagina protects the uterus, or womb. It is tightly closed during pregnancy and blocked by a plug of mucus, which is expelled as, or shortly before, labor begins. The cervix then stretches to allow the baby through.

Uterus: a pear-shaped, hollow organ at the top of the vagina, which provides a safe environment for the fetus to develop within.

Fallopian tubes: two tubes, one on each side of the uterus, which lead from the ovaries to the uterus. Fertilization occurs here.

Ovary: an almond-shaped organ at the end of each fallopian tube on either side of the pelvic cavity, responsible for releasing eggs and for manufacturing sex hormones.

take notes

You can help your caregivers help you by keeping good records. Note any symptoms, issues, or questions that arise during your pregnancy on the blank pages provided at the end of each of the three sections in this book. Bring this book to medical appointments, so you can discuss your progress in full.

hormones & ovulation

A handful of hormones play an active role during ovulation and subsequent pregnancy.

Every month, your brain releases gonadotropin-releasing hormone (GnRH), which triggers the pituitary gland, a pea-sized gland located at the base of your brain, to produce two sex hormones: follicle-stimulating hormone (FSH) and luteinizing hormone (LH). These natural chemical messengers are sent to the ovaries, where FSH helps an egg to develop and LH helps stimulate ovulation.

Once you are pregnant, human chorionic gonadotropin (hCG) is produced to stimulate the hormones progesterone and estrogen so that the pregnancy can be sustained until the placenta is developed enough to take over this job.

Estrogen, released by the ovaries, helps provide a proper environment for the fetus by causing the lining of the uterus to thicken so that it can support the

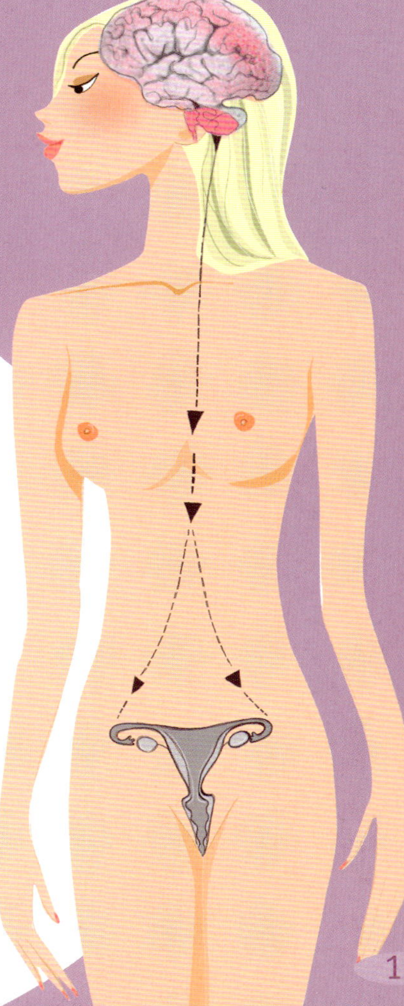

fetus. Estrogen maintains the placenta so that oxygen and nutrients can pass from the mother to the fetus. It also stimulates the development of most fetal organs, and regulates the fetus's bone density.

Without progesterone, your pregnancy could not be maintained. Progesterone, together with another hormone called relaxin, prevents early miscarriage caused by uterine contractions. It also prevents lactation during pregnancy by inhibiting the action of prolactin (see below).

Once you go into labor, your body releases oxytocin, which helps to dilate the cervix prior to birth, causes contractions during labor, and releases milk during breast-feeding. Following the birth, prolactin is responsible for stimulating the flow of milk through the breasts.

preparing to conceive

Once you have decided to get pregnant, examine your lifestyle and change any unhealthy habits. There are steps you can take prior to conception to help foster a successful pregnancy and produce a healthy baby. If your pregnancy was unplanned, make any necessary changes as soon as you know you are pregnant.

do's and don'ts

Mothers-to-be face an ever-growing list of don'ts, from the proven offenders—cigarettes, drugs, and alcohol—to the questionable or unproven—hair dye, acrylic nails, tanning beds, underwire bras, and Botox. It's not easy, but a sensible plan ought to include limiting exposure to harsh chemicals and environments, and discussing issues and questions with your obstetrician.

experts recommend that you:

Maintain an average body weight for your height.

Exercise regularly to improve your cardiovascular condition and muscle tone.

Eat nutritious meals with an optimal balance of carbohydrates, protein, and fat and adequate amounts of folic acid, C and B vitamins, calcium, magnesium, and iron.

Stop smoking (if you are smoker) and ask others not to smoke around you. Also avoid alcohol and caffeine.

Avoid using medications other than those prescribed or recommended by your doctor.

Have a physical checkup to discuss any problems that could adversely impact your pregnancy, such as diabetes or high blood pressure. If you are over 35, review any age-related concerns with your doctor.

Have a dental exam but avoid X-rays or dental work if you suspect you are already pregnant.

Sign up for a prenatal class.

Review your family history with your doctor and ask if you should meet with a genetic counselor.

Let your caregivers know if you have an ongoing medical problem or are on medication—many common medications can cause problems prior to conception or during pregnancy.

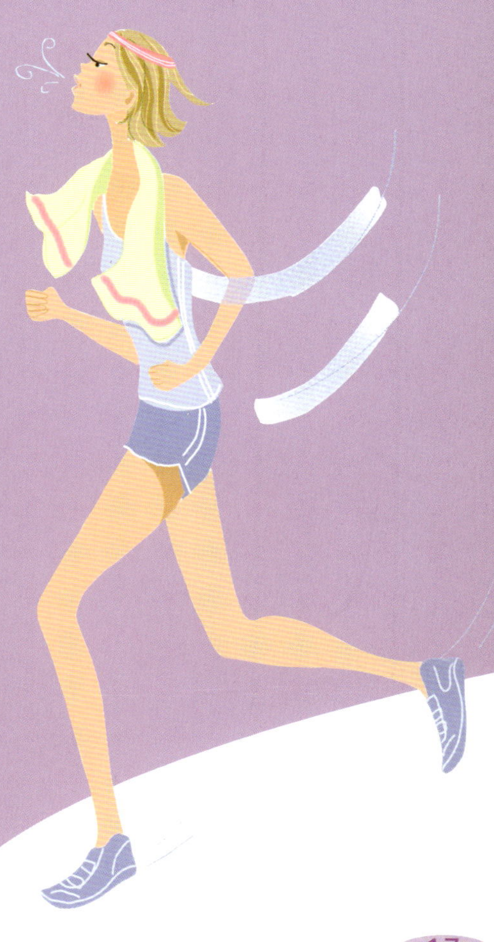

preparing to conceive

Once you become pregnant, a healthy balance of vitamins and minerals will be extremely important. Begin building your reserves before you conceive. While it's true that you can obtain most of the nutrition you need from a healthy diet (see p. 89), many women find it difficult to plan, shop for, and cook every meal due to their hectic lifestyles. If this is the case for you, then you might want to consider taking a vitamin supplement.

prenatal vitamin formulas

Simply taking more of your regular vitamins could be dangerous. For example, the quantity of vitamin A in many standard formulas can cause birth defects. Instead, choose a formula that has been specially designed for pregnant women.

Folate-friendly foods include asparagus; leafy green vegetables; citrus fruits and juices; beans; peanuts; broccoli; peas; lentils; whole grains.

what do you need?

Iron helps to prevent anemia.

Folic acid and zinc help prevent birth defects. Zinc also helps prevent fetal immune deficiencies and abnormal behavior in children.

Calcium helps maintain the mother's bone density and supports the growth of fetal bones.

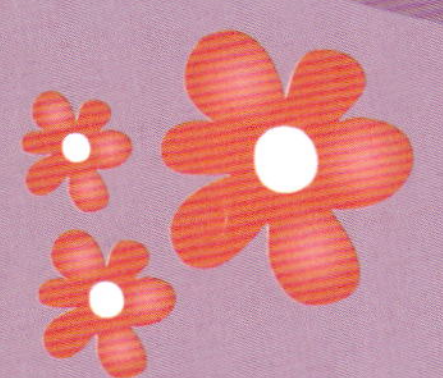

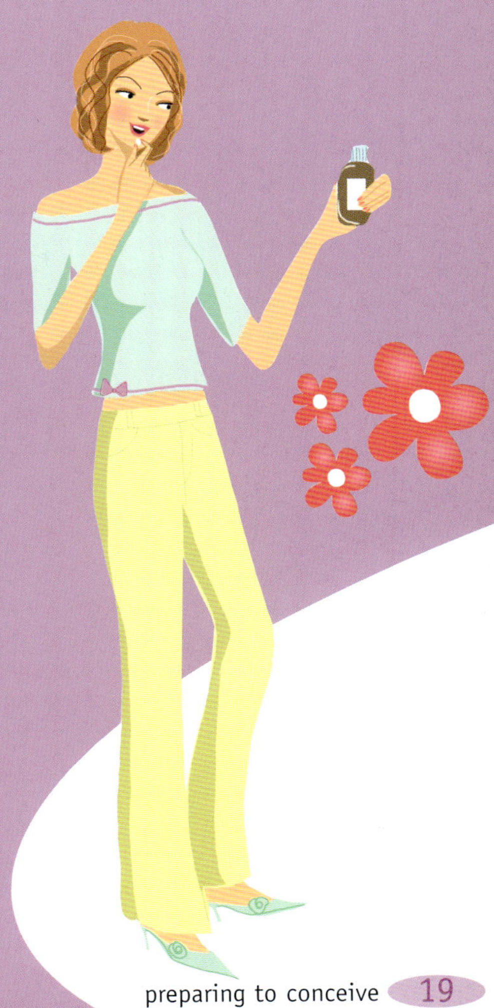

nature's helper—folic acid

Folic acid is a B vitamin that helps to prevent birth defects of the brain and spinal cord, but only if it is taken prior to conception and during the first few weeks of pregnancy. All women of childbearing age are urged to take a multivitamin that contains between 400 and 600 micrograms (μg) of folic acid every day and to eat a diet rich in foods that contain folate or folic acid.

vitamin a alert

The body makes its own vitamin A from beta-carotene, which is found in yellow, orange, and green vegetables, and you should not be tempted to increase your intake of vitamin A beyond the minimum requirements. At least one study has shown that high doses of vitamin A can double the risk of having a baby with birth defects. Foods that contain high quantities of vitamin A such as beef liver, eggs, dairy products, and fortified breakfast cereals should be eaten in moderation.

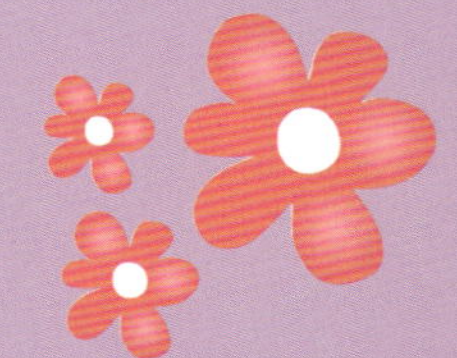

the magic of conception

Conception is essentially a two-stage process. First, the sperm has to fertilize the egg, then the egg has to implant successfully in the uterus.

fertilization

Within your ovaries are a number of follicles, each one containing an egg. Once a month an egg matures and is released from its follicle into your fallopian tube. It then moves on toward your uterus. In a typical 28-day menstrual cycle, this process—ovulation—occurs around day 14. When the egg reaches the outer third of the fallopian tube, it meets up with sperm that have been propelled up the vagina following ejaculation. Only one sperm will penetrate the outer surface of the egg. When this occurs, the nuclei of the egg and the sperm unite, forming a zygote (fertilized egg).

when is the best time to conceive?

Once an egg is released from your ovary, it will survive for a maximum of 24 hours. Your partner's sperm loses its ability to fertilize an egg some 24 to 36 hours after ejaculation. For the best chances of conception, therefore, sexual intercourse should take place one day before, or just after, ovulation.

one baby or two?

Around 1 in 80 pregnancies results in twins, and women over the age of 35 are more likely to have them. Around two-thirds of twins are non-identical, and are the result of two eggs being released by the ovaries and fertilized by different sperm. Identical twins result from one fertilized egg splitting in two.

what determines my baby's gender?

Gender is determined by two chromosomes (labelled "X" and "Y"). Females, and all of the eggs females produce, have two X chromosomes. Males have one X and one Y chromosome. Sperm have either an X or a Y chromosome. If a sperm with an X chromosome fertilizes an egg, the baby will be a girl (XX). If a Y sperm fertilizes an egg, it will be a boy (XY).

Of the 200 to 400 million sperm deposited in the vagina during the typical male ejaculation, fewer than 200 make it as far as the released egg.

the magic of conception

The second stage of conception—when the fertilized egg implants in the womb—puts you on the road to having a baby.

implantation

Following conception, your fertilized egg begins its journey down the fallopian tube to your womb. This journey takes about three to five days. Within 24 hours, the cell divides into two, then continues to divide as it travels on to the uterus. By the fourth day after fertilization, there will be more than 100 cells in all. They organize themselves in two layers around a fluid-filled bubble, forming an early-stage embryo called a blastocyst.

Meanwhile, stimulated by the hormone progesterone, the uterine lining has been growing thick and abundant with blood vessels in preparation for implantation. Seven to nine days after fertilization, the blastocyst begins to embed itself in the uterine wall. By day nine it is fully covered, and implantation is complete.

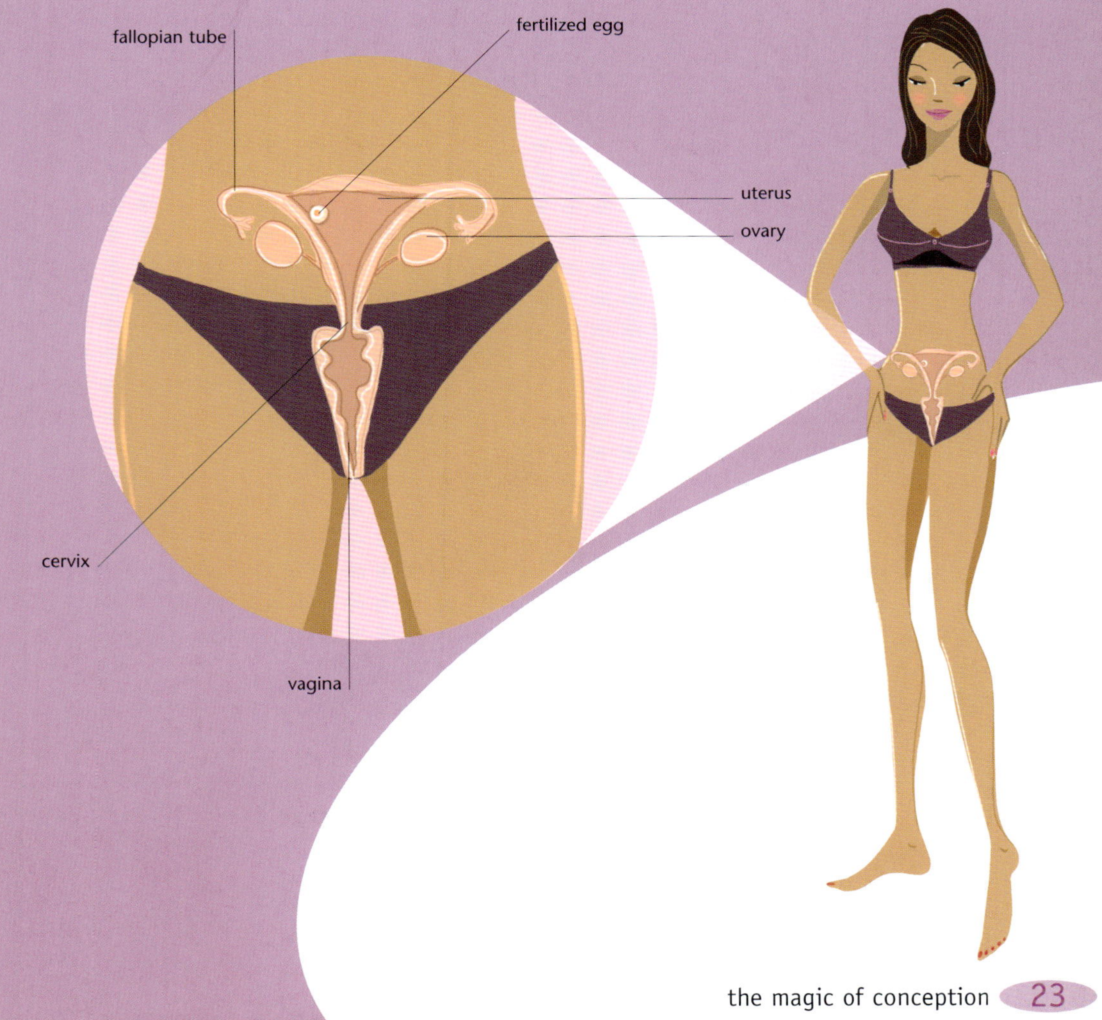
fallopian tube
fertilized egg
uterus
ovary
cervix
vagina

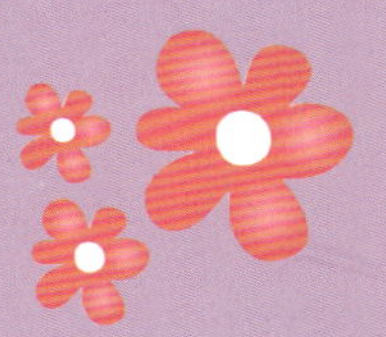

signs of pregnancy

Some women claim to have known that they were pregnant from the moment of conception. Others do not begin to suspect until several weeks into their pregnancy, when they start to experience dizziness, nausea, or extreme fatigue. These, along with missing your next period—some two weeks after fertilization—are common signs that you are pregnant.

what to look out for

Frequent urination: as early as one week after conception, you may notice a need to pass urine more often than usual, because the swelling uterus puts pressure on your bladder.

Large and tender breasts: your breasts will swell within the first few weeks of pregnancy—even before you miss your next period—and your nipples may also become slightly larger and darker.

A change in food preferences: you'll find yourself rejecting certain foods and drinks—sometimes even the smell of them will be enough to put you off.

Strange taste: many women notice a "metallic" taste in the mouth from early on.

Fatigue: you may find yourself overcome with tiredness during the first few weeks of your pregnancy; at times you may also feel faint or dizzy.

Nausea or vomiting: many, but not all, women experience "morning sickness" from about the sixth week. It is unusual for symptoms to last beyond the first trimester.

Moodiness: it is normal to experience mood swings early on, from ecstatic highs to tearful lows and everything in between.

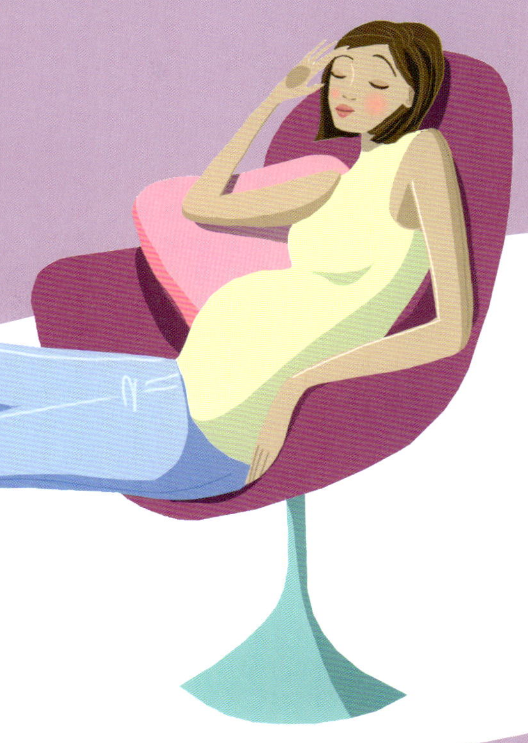

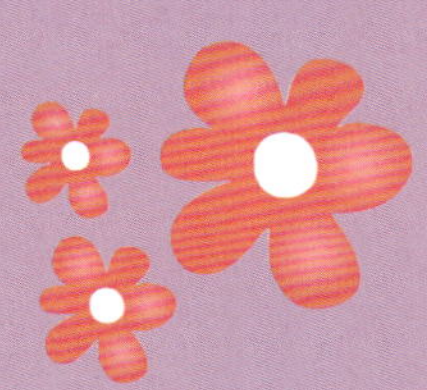

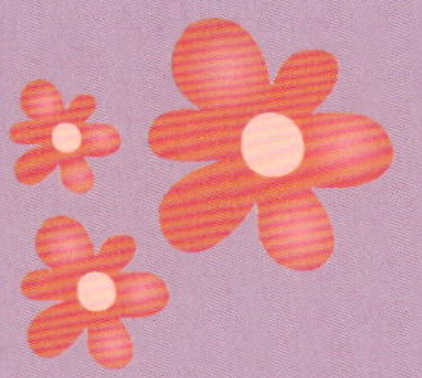

confirming your pregnancy

There are several different kinds of pregnancy tests available, most of which work on the same principle. They are designed to detect hCG, a hormone that becomes elevated in the urine and the blood of pregnant women. The level of this hormone increases dramatically after implantation, reaching peak levels 70 days after the last menstrual period.

If you suspect that you are pregnant but a test proves negative, repeat it in a couple of days. If you are pregnant, the levels of hCG will be higher. Most kits contain two tests for this reason. False negatives are not uncommon, but a positive test result means that you really are pregnant.

Almost all tests are carried out on a urine sample, and it is important to make sure you use the first urine of the

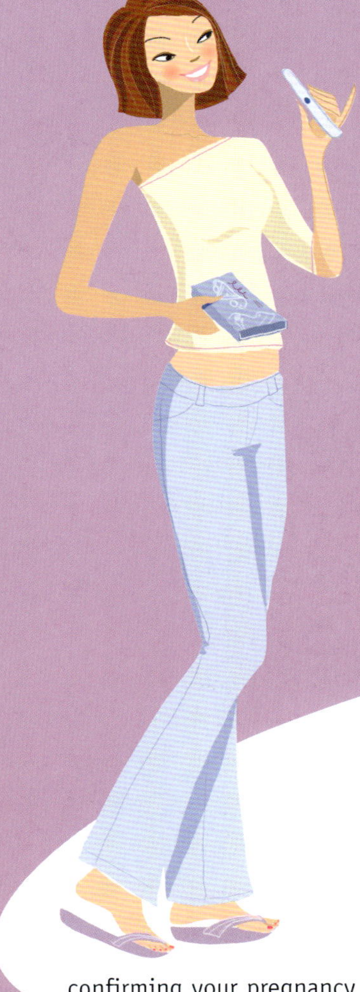

day, when levels of hCG will be most concentrated. Although some tests can detect pregnancy as early as 24 hours after the implantation of the fertilized egg, others are not as sensitive. If you are using a home-testing kit, it is best to wait until at least two days after you miss your period in order to guarantee maximum reliability (most kits offer 95 percent accuracy). If the test is negative, but your period doesn't start when it should, repeat the test.

Although a positive test is a strong indicator that you are pregnant, you should visit your doctor for confirmation and to get booked in for prenatal care, which starts early in your pregnancy. This is also a good time to discuss birth options and to pick up any relevant leaflets.

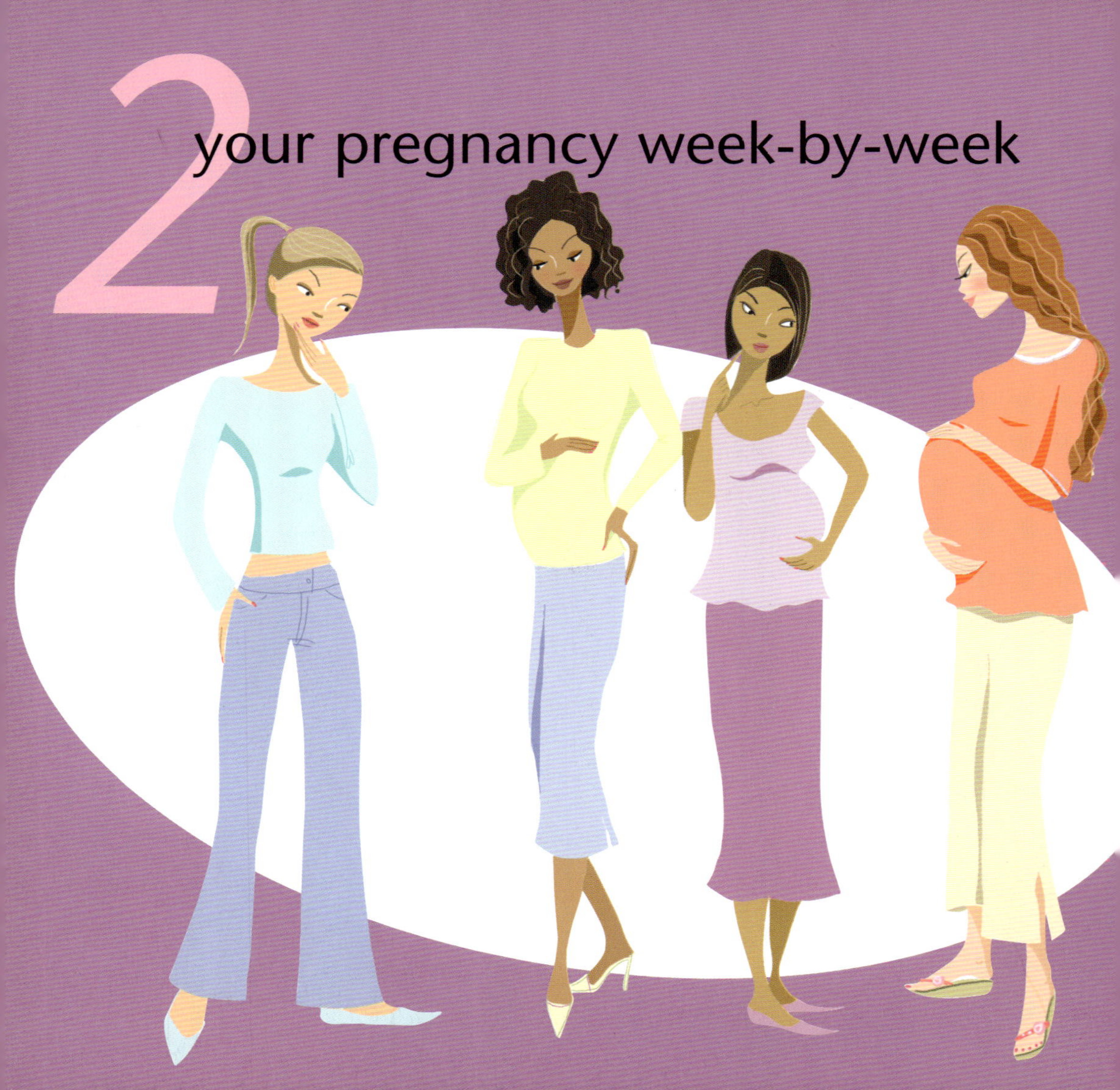

2 your pregnancy week-by-week

This section tells you all there is to know about your baby's development from week one through birth. You'll also learn what to expect physically during each trimester as your body changes to accommodate first the embryo, and then the growing fetus. There are also journal pages for you to record your thoughts and feelings as your pregnancy advances as well as questions for healthcare providers. Take the book with you to all your prenatal visits and share the details of your experience with your healthcare providers, asking any questions you might have.

first trimester

you

the stages of pregnancy

Pregnancy is usually described as consisting of three trimesters, each lasting three months and associated with a major aspect of your baby's development.

- First trimester: cell differentiation from the fertilized egg
- Second trimester: the major development of basic body systems in the fetus
- Third trimester: growth to a mature fetus capable of life outside the mother's womb

when is my baby due?

Typically, a baby's birth date is calculated by counting 280 days (40 weeks) from the first day of the mother's last menstrual period (LMP) to the time of birth. This is often educated guesswork, as many women do not have a precise recollection of when their last menstrual period began.

your baby

pre-embryonic stage

Fertilization of the egg occurs during the second week, and the fertilized egg is fully implanted in the wall of the uterus by the end of week three.

Between days 24 and 28, the rapidly multiplying cells in the embryo begin to form three separate layers, each with different characteristics and functions.

- Endoderm: this will become, among other things, your baby's gastrointestinal tract and endocrine glands
- Ectoderm: this will become your baby's skin and nervous system
- Mesoderm: this will develop into your baby's connective tissue, circulatory system, skeleton, and muscles

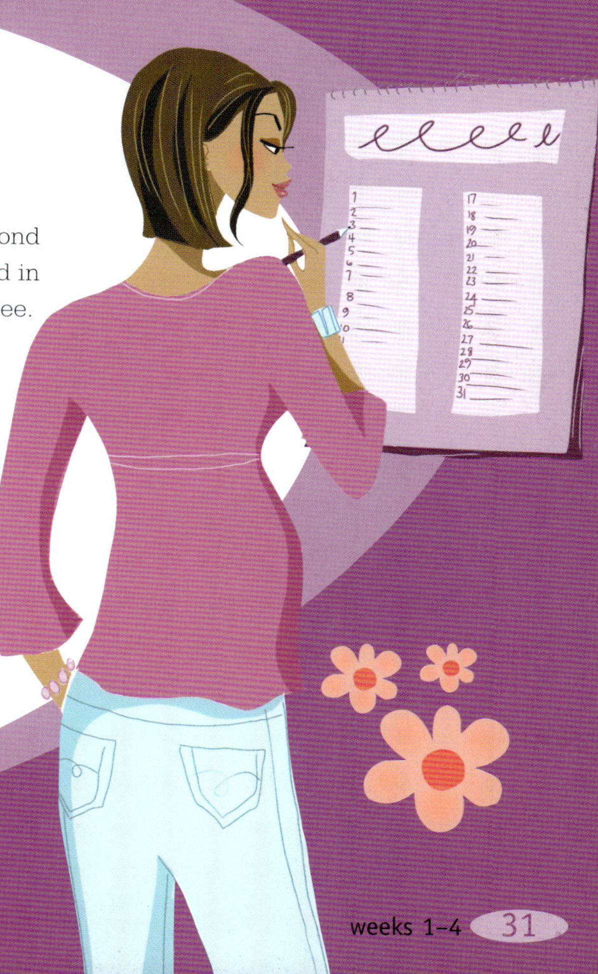

first trimester

you

what's happening to me?

No matter how much you've longed for a child or how far in advance you've planned, you probably still don't know what to expect from this pregnancy. You may have fears and doubts or worries about whether you will be able to carry the fetus to term. You may feel the first stirrings of anxiety at the thought of how your life will change. What kind of a mother will you be? If you have a partner, you may wonder how he feels about the big event or his role in family life. If you have concerns such as these, remember that you are not alone. Most mothers-to-be are apprehensive, especially the first time around. Take a deep breath and relax.

how do I look?

Most of the changes during the first trimester are internal. Your doctor will note changes in your pelvis. Your cervix becomes softer and, as its blood supply increases, its color changes to a shade of purple. The area between the cervix and the uterus also softens.

your baby

early organ development

During week five, specialized cells develop that will become your baby's brain, heart, kidneys, thyroid, spinal cord, stomach, intestines, and other organs. Ectodermic cells on the back of the embryo form a groove and then fold in to create the neural tube, which will eventually become the brain and spinal cord. Another tube-like structure forms a rudimentary gastrointestinal tract, including a working liver. By day 31, blood begins to circulate through a third tubular structure—a primitive heart—attached to the outside of the embryo's body. The placenta is in the process of evolving. Facial features begin to appear: indentations mark the start of ears, eyes, and a nose.

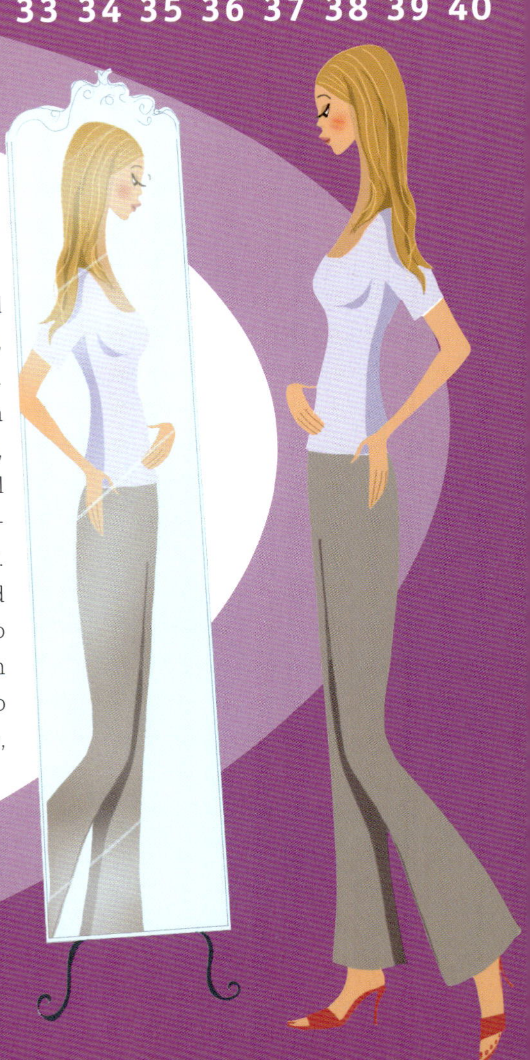

first trimester

you

how do you feel?

Rising hormone levels cause your breasts to enlarge in preparation for milk production. The areola and nipple change color and veins beneath the skin become more visible as the blood supply to the breasts increases. Expect your breasts, and nipples in particular, to feel tender. A bra designed for pregnant women offers extra support and greater comfort, and will be an essential item of clothing as the pregnancy progresses.

your baby

limb buds and more

The organs continue to develop. The neural tube closes at either end: the front part of the tube becomes the brain and the back part becomes the spinal cord. All along the embryo's back, ridges start to appear that will eventually become the spinal column and vertebrae. Buds of tissue mark the beginnings of arms and legs. A rudimentary mouth forms, and the jaws start to take shape. The esophagus, trachea (windpipe), stomach, and intestines continue to form. The ducts of pancreas and liver begin to grow. The Eustachian tubes form now, along with the middle ear cavity and the tonsils. By the end of this week, at 42 days, the embryo has a heartbeat. The tubular heart is busy pumping primitive red blood cells through the major blood vessels. The placenta has begun to function.

life-support system

Once it is fully functioning, the placenta works as an exchange system, taking oxygen and nutrients from your bloodstream, filtering them, and passing them via the umbilical cord to your baby. All your baby's waste, including carbon dioxide, crosses the placenta into your body for disposal.

first trimester

you

how do you feel?

In the early weeks and months, minor discomforts, such as wanting to urinate often, can start to get you down.

frequent urination

The uterus puts pressure on the bladder, so you will feel the urge to urinate more often. You may even leak urine while laughing or sneezing. Keep hydrated by drinking eight glasses of water a day, but avoid drinking at night so you can get uninterrupted sleep. By month four, when the uterus has shifted, the urge to urinate so much should decrease.

vaginal discharge

Increased estrogen levels trigger mucus production, resulting in a thick, whitish, acidic discharge called leukorrhea. You can alleviate the symptoms by bathing often and wearing loose cotton panties. White or yellowish discharge may also indicate yeast infection. Pregnancy can also disrupt the body's natural defenses against the overgrowth of *Candida albicans* (a natural organism that grows in the vagina), resulting in a yeast infection.

your baby

the developing nervous system

The embryo's nervous system becomes more refined. Now there is a brain with 10 nerve pairs and five areas of specialized cells. Nerves also appear in the newly forming muscles. Fat cells are present, too. The circulatory system continues to develop. The tubular heart divides into two distinct chambers.

On the "face" of the embryo, depressions marking the eyes and the nostrils continue to deepen. Arm and leg buds start to elongate. By the end of the week, paddle-shaped appendages appear at the end of the limb buds. These are embryonic hands and feet. The embryo is sometimes said to resemble a shrimp: curved like the letter "C," with a tail at one end and a big head at the other.

Your developing baby is now between a quarter and one-third of an inch long.

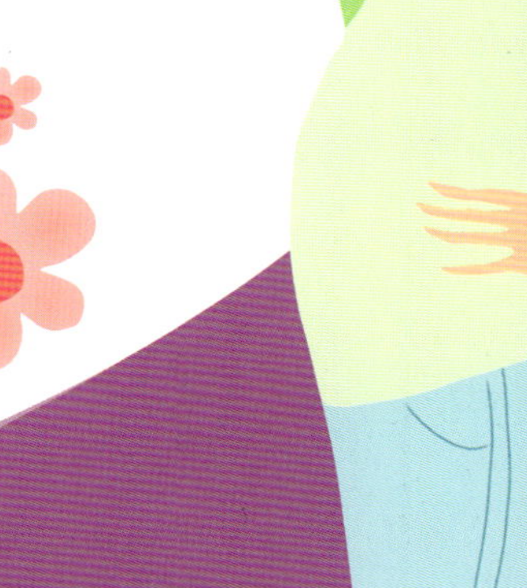

first trimester

you

i feel terrible

Many expectant mothers experience nausea and vomiting during the first trimester. This has been linked to a rise in the level of the hormone human chorionic gonadotrophin (hCG), which regulates the body's supply of estrogen and progesterone during pregnancy. This is often referred to as "morning sickness," but it can occur at any time. The box on the right details some tips for dealing with it.

your baby

a flexible skeleton

The nose and mouth become more distinct, and the upper lip appears. The three parts of the ear—external, middle, and interna—are present. The jaws start to turn to bone. A skeleton forms. For the most part, it's made of cartilage, a flexible, semitransparent tissue that is the precursor to bone. The arms are now slightly bowed where the elbows are growing, and there are webbed toes and fingers on the feet and hands. Muscles continue to develop, including the chambered heart. The liver is far enough along to start manufacturing a variety of blood cells. In addition to the trachea, there are the elementary bronchial tubes and two lung buds. Sex glands start forming. The tail is smaller than it was last week; over the next few weeks it will gradually disappear.

At just under a half inch in size, your developing baby is almost twice as big as it was last week.

morning sickness

- Avoid foods and smells that trigger nausea: greasy foods, coffee, and cigarette smoke
- Increase the number of times you eat during the day
- Drink water or other fluids between mealtimes
- Snack on carbonated drinks and crackers or dry toast

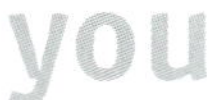

you

the first prenatal appointment

Around weeks 8 to 12, you will attend your first appointment at the prenatal clinic for a full checkup.

Your doctor or midwife will assess your health in order to determine how your pregnancy will progress. You will be asked questions about your and your partner's medical history, and you will probably have lots of questions of your own to ask the nurse or midwife.

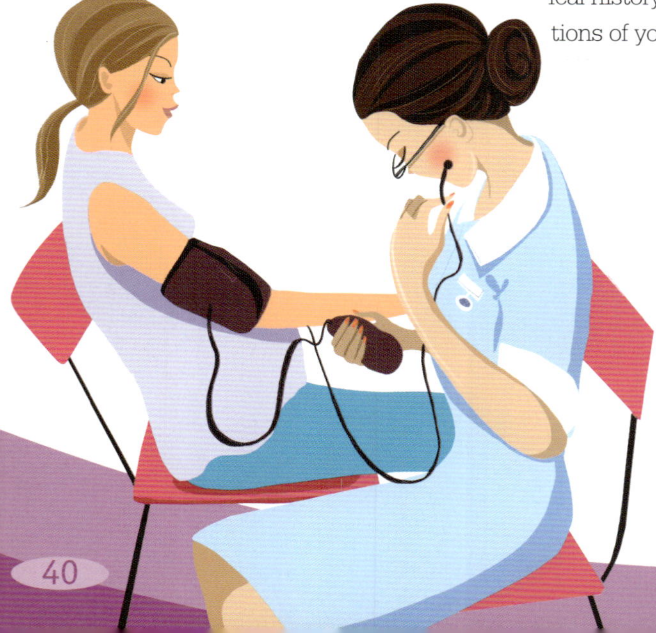

typical tests

- Blood test: to determine blood group; to find your hemoglobin level; to check for immunity to rubella; to check for anemia
- Urine test: to check for kidney infection; to monitor sugar levels
- Breast examination: to check condition and for any lumps
- Hair, nails, teeth, eyes: to detect any dietary deficiencies
- Blood pressure: to check if raised

common questions to expect

- Are there any illnesses which are common in your families?
- Have you or your partner ever been seriously ill?
- Is this your first pregnancy?
- Have your ever miscarried?
- What is your menstrual history?

questions I want to ask at this appointment

based on the questions on the left, note here anything, however trivial it may seem, that might be relevant to your pregnancy

you

a word about miscarriage

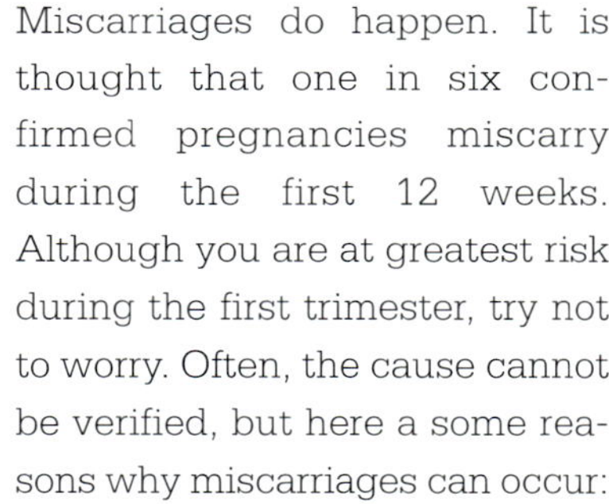

Miscarriages do happen. It is thought that one in six confirmed pregnancies miscarry during the first 12 weeks. Although you are at greatest risk during the first trimester, try not to worry. Often, the cause cannot be verified, but here a some reasons why miscarriages can occur:

- The embryo may have a defect that would prevent it from developing normally
- You may have an incompetent cervix—that is, it fails to remain closed
- You and your partner may have incompatible blood types
- The placenta may fail to develop properly
- Certain medications—aspirin, for example—are believed to cause miscarriage

what to do

A miscarriage usually starts with bleeding. It can be light or heavy, and might be accompanied by abdominal pain. If you think you are miscarrying, you must contact your doctor, who will ask you a number of questions in order to assess the situation and advise you on what to do next. This may involve either going to the hospital or lying flat at home to see if the bleeding stops. You will also be advised to try to keep any blood clots for examination.

your baby

becoming human in appearance

By the ninth week, some essential parts of your developing baby's anatomy are recognizable. The head and limbs are growing more distinct. Toes are developing at the ends of the feet, and there is a discernible bump for the nose. The eyes are moving closer together, away from the sides of the head and toward the front of the face. There is a distinct mouth and tongue forming in the front of the face.

Internally, the chambered heart is beating, the stomach is distinct in the middle of the body, and the last part of the large intestine, the rectum, has formed. Reproductive and urinary organs, including the bladder, are forming, and the testes and ovaries begin to differentiate.

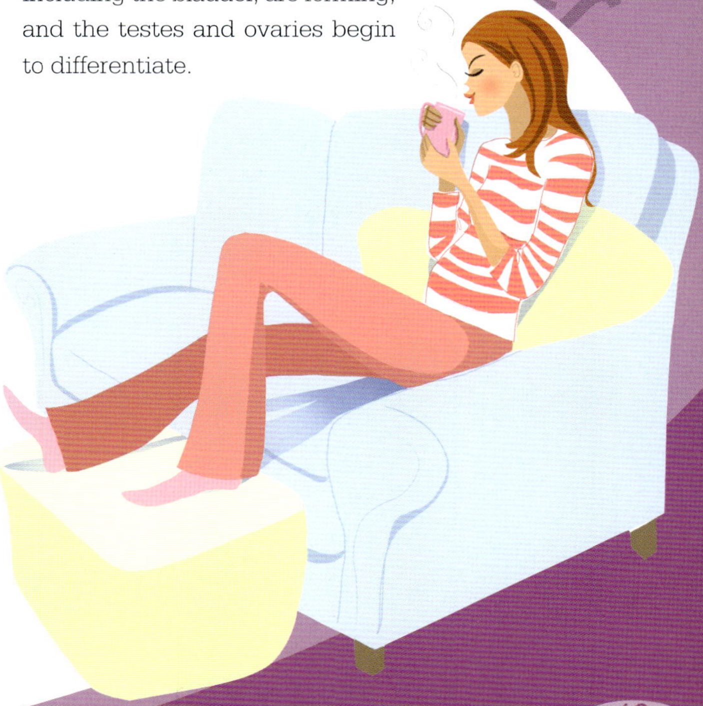

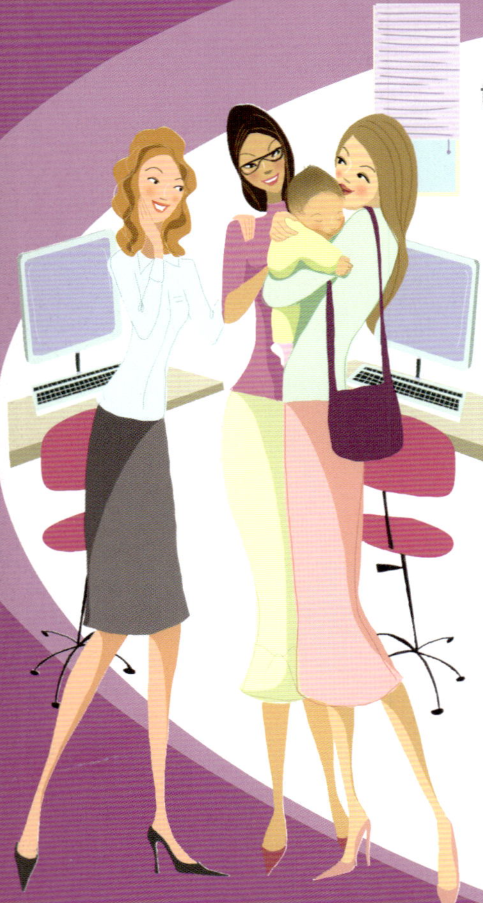

you

thinking ahead: career plans

It is never too soon to consider your career options. At this stage, you should be feeling good. Look honestly at how having a baby will affect your work in the year ahead, and consider the expectations you have of yourself and your partner. Share your feelings and concerns with your partner and be equally willing to have him share his feelings with you. Start figuring out how you will handle any necessary changes together. You may find the following questions useful:

- Will you need a daycare provider?
- Will you need to postpone any promotion or career move?
- Will your partner need to work longer hours, or take a more stressful or time-consuming job to make up for your lost income?
- How will your decision to work affect your view of yourself as a mother?
- How will your decision to stay home affect your self-esteem?

your baby

good-bye embryo, hello fetus

By the end of the tenth week, the embryo has become a fetus with facial features, external ears, and lips. The tiny skeleton of cartilage is lengthening and hardening into bone in places. Circulation is well-established through the heart and umbilical cord. External genitalia appear now, and the fetus can be recognized as a boy or a girl for the first time. The lower end of the rectal passage opens to create the anus. Muscles grow in the arms, legs, trunk, and head. The larger muscles are able to contract now, and the fetus may even start to be able to move, although too slowly for you to feel it yet.

Your developing baby is a little bigger than an inch.

first trimester

you

the first ultrasound

Toward the end of your first trimester, you will be booked in for an ultrasound scan. This five-minute procedure examines the baby in your uterus, and confirms the fetus's age. You will need a full bladder. A warm jelly is spread over your abdomen and the ultrasound equipment passed over it. This sends back signals that can then be seen on a monitor.

pregnancy highs: that's my baby

Ultrasound works by converting the echoes of sound waves into pictures as they bounce off different parts of the fetus's body. What you see is a photographic image of the baby in your womb. This is often an extremely emotional experience because you are getting your first actual glimpse of your baby.

what's on the scan

The most important thing that you will see on the ultrasound is the baby's heart beating, which will show as a pulsing light. The technician will also be able to point out the head and the curve of the spine. Arms and legs may be less clear, but you might be able to see them, too.

questions I want to ask the technician

note down anything that seems important to ask, such as do you want to know the baby's sex?

you

how are you feeling?

self-help for fatigue

- Go to bed earlier
- Take moderate exercise in the fresh air
- Ease back on personal commitments and activities
- Lower your expectations for taking care of the house
- Seek help from family members or professionals
- Take frequent naps

You may be experiencing a few minor problems at this stage. Increased amounts of estrogen can cause your nose to get congested, which may lead to headaches. Also, as the number of blood vessels in your nose increases, you may get more nosebleeds. Temporary relief may be found by using a vaporizer that emits cool moisture into the air. Alternatively, apply warm compresses to the face.

i'm exhausted

Fatigue is one of the first signs of pregnancy. During the first few weeks in particular, you will find yourself needing increasingly early nights. Try to conserve energy by adopting the habits listed on the left.

your baby

external refinements

The fetus now has a profile with a protruding nose and a bulbous forehead. Eyelids fuse shut. The lips separate from the jaw and can move in a sucking motion. Inside the mouth, buds of tissue mark the beginnings of teeth. Limbs are growing more proportional. The arms are more developed than the legs, and the tiny fingers can fold into a fist. Nails start forming on fingers and toes.

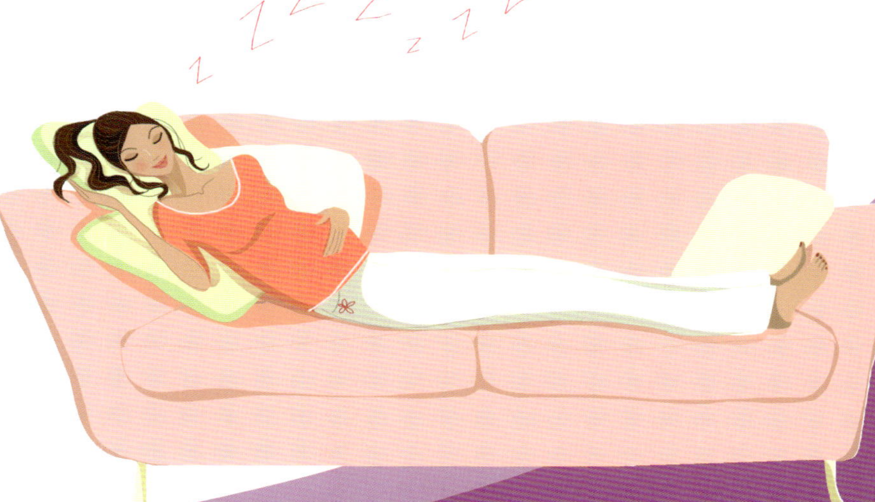

first trimester

you

thinking ahead: health insurance

By the end of week 14, your developing baby is about 4½ inches long from the top of the head to the bottom of its foot. The head makes up almost half of this total length.

Review your medical benefits plan to find out what expenses it covers. Ask about:

- Prenatal care
- Prenatal tests
- Anesthesia
- Delivery options
- Emergency cesarean sections (C-sections)
- What deductibles you're expected to pay and what your total out-of-pocket expenses are likely to be
- Which hospitals are covered
- Whether it covers complementary health care, such as a midwife or massage therapist
- How to go about adding your baby to the plan and the kind of coverage you can expect for him or her

your baby

internal refinements

About this time, males start producing testosterone. The bladder has formed, and the fetus can urinate. The liver is now producing most of the red blood cells. The thyroid produces hormones, too. The lungs are formed. The brain has differentiated into left and right halves.

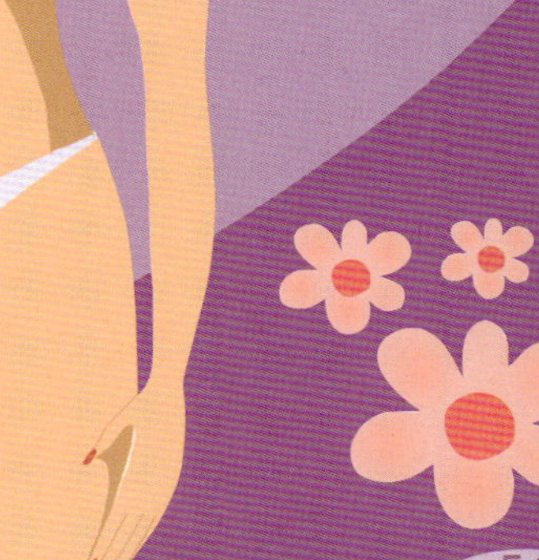

you

strengthen your relationship

Don't forget that your partner has concerns, too. He has to cope with your mood swings and may feel at a loss when it comes to figuring out how to help you. He may become more, or less, attentive, depending on how stressed he feels about the responsibility of bringing a child into the world. It is not unusual for a partner to worry about being a good provider. Some feel left out of the process as friends and family focus more attention on the mother. Make this a positive time for the two of you by giving each other lots of mutual support, and have fun planning this next phase of your life together. If you want your relationship to grow stronger, you need to be in tune with each other:

- Encourage one another to talk about the way you feel
- Involve your partner in all your baby-related appointments
- Discuss your partner's likely role once the baby is born
- Take time off together, such as nights out or weekend breaks

your partner

thinking ahead: maternity/paternity leave

Find out what your company's maternity and paternity leave policy is. Some states have laws establishing how long a mother may take a leave of absence from a job without pay and still expect to retain her position. Although it is rare to take actual paid maternity leave, you will probably be able to cover the time you take off by using a combination of short-term disability, sick leave, unpaid leave, and vacation time. According to the Family and Medical Leave Act (FMLA), covered employers must grant an eligible employee up to 12 work weeks unpaid leave during any 12-month period for the birth and care of the newborn child. For details and to check your eligibility, visit the U.S. Department of Labor's web site, *www.dol.gov*.

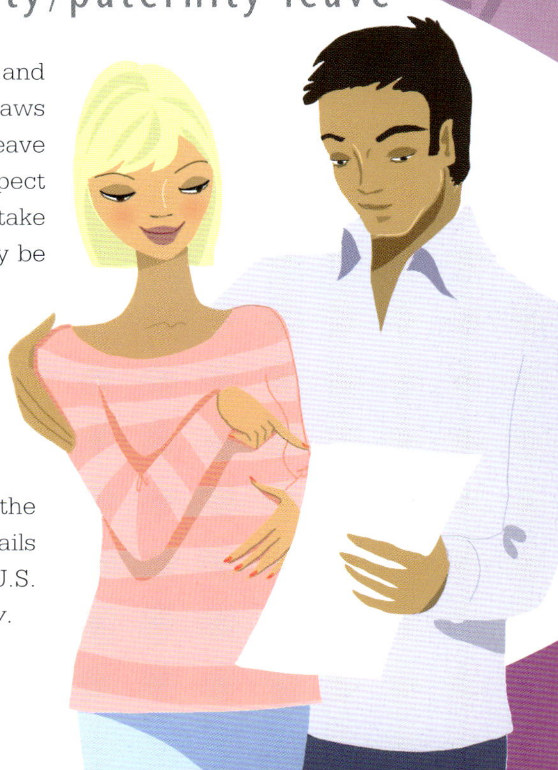

my thoughts and feelings—use this page to sum up how you feel after three months; what will you tell your baby about this time?

questions I want to ask at my next appointment

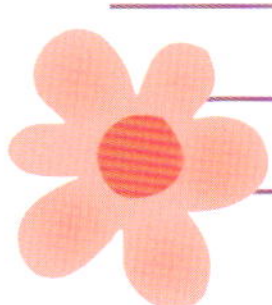

second trimester

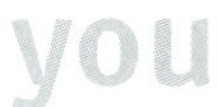

you

what's happening to me?

There's no denying that you are pregnant now. Your pregnancy is becoming visible on the outside, too, as the uterus starts to bulge just above your pubic bone. Your clothes are starting to get tight. It's time to go shopping for maternity outfits. Your body image starts to change, and you may feel embarrassed or incredibly proud about your new status.

how do I feel?

Many of the physical difficulties experienced during the first trimester start to subside and your energy returns. Most women enjoy the second trimester the most, since they feel less nauseous than they did in the first trimester and aren't as big as they will be in the third trimester.

your baby

all in place

Inside your womb, the fetus is starting to look human, all the major organs are working, and the heart is beating about twice as fast as yours is. It is possible that you will feel those first movements, known as the "quickening," early in this trimester, although most first-time moms are not conscious of them until some weeks later. Urge your partner to feel the baby. Your baby has been floating around freely for weeks now, but you are not conscious of this as the baby is cushioned in the amniotic fluid. Once it is larger, the uterus will start to press against your abdomen and you will feel movement.

pregnancy highs: daydreaming

At about this time your feelings toward the growing baby may start to change. You will start to realize that your unborn child is separate from you, and is a person in its own right. This is exciting, and you may find yourself becoming even more preoccupied with plans for the future. You may spend time daydreaming about what your baby, and then child, will look like or grow up to be. Your partner, on the other hand, may already be visualizing the fetus as a small child of six or seven.

you

mutual uncertainty

You may feel a greater need for your partner to demonstrate affection, but your mood swings, and the reality of increasing responsibilities may make your partner withdraw a bit. He has a lot to think about, too. Perhaps you can encourage him to find a creative outlet such as working on the baby's room, or to find a new hobby as a distraction. Realize that this situation is perfectly normal, even if it is a bit stressful, and it will not be long before the two of you reconnect as your pregnancy reaches the last (third) trimester.

- Keep talking: accept that you are both in this together
- Try to see each other's points of view
- Realize that this is a temporary time, and treasure it
- Spend time together—take a long walk, cook a special meal, go to the movies

second trimester

your baby

a growth spurt

Now that all the major organs are in place, the body starts to grow larger. As the limbs become more proportional to the body, they increase in flexibility. Arms bend at the elbows. Legs bend at the knees. The fetus can stretch, move its head, wrists, hands, feet, and toes. Posture also improves as the muscles and skeleton continue to develop.

second trimester

you

let's shop

Now you have reached the stage where you have a noticeable bump, many of your pre-pregnant clothes will no longer fit properly, if at all. This is great news, because it means you can go out shopping, but don't rush into anything without thinking things through. You are not going to be this size for very long and you will get bigger. You need to find ways of making your clothes last for the months to come. Here are some tips:

- Buy clothes one size up to get the most wear out of them
- Choose garments with built-in elastic for expansion
- Opt for stretchy fabrics for maximum comfort
- Raid your partner's closet for loose shirts and sweaters
- Make sure you invest in good, supportive underwear

your baby

boy or girl?

Your baby's gender was determined at the time of conception and the internal and external genitals have been developing for some weeks now. But around this time, they are visible on a further ultrasound scan, as long as the fetus is facing in the right direction. A skilled technician can tell the sex and will tell you, if you want to know. Most first-time parents can't "read" an ultrasound well enough—it would need to be pointed out to you. If your baby is a girl, by about this time the follicles that hold all the eggs she'll ever have—about six million—are in place.

pregnancy lows: constipation

High levels of progesterone, uterine pressure on the intestine, and a slackening in muscle tone contribute to sluggish bowel movements. A poor diet or iron supplements (however necessary) can also lead to constipation at this time. To combat the problem, drink plenty of water and eat a diet rich in fiber. Your care provider might recommend a fiber supplement or stool softener, but do not be tempted to take strong laxatives.

At 18 weeks, your developing baby is almost 6 inches long and weighs about 7 ounces.

you

changes to your skin

Starting mid-pregnancy, your skin may go through a number of changes, many of which are caused by the increased levels of certain hormones. Here are the three most common developments, although they do not affect all women.

Stretch marks: the high level of sex hormones in your body can have an effect on the collagen in your skin, leaving it thin and stretched in areas. The most likely affected areas are breasts, thighs, and abdomen. You cannot prevent stretch marks, but you can help your skin from feeling dried out or itchy by applying vitamin E cream, cocoa butter, and other types of mild oil such as baby oil or almond oil.

Linea nigra: a dark line down the center of the abdomen may begin from around the fourteenth week of pregnancy. This is due to an increase in the production of the pigment melanin. It will fade after the birth.

Pigmentation: dark patches on the skin, known as chloasma, may appear. These should disappear once pregnancy is over. Consider wearing some sunscreen on your face, since exposure to the sun can increase pigmentation.

your baby

skin deep

Hair grows on top of the head and fine hair, called "lanugo," appears on the body. This may play some role in temperature regulation, and usually disappears before the birth (premature babies may be born with traces remaining). Sweat glands start to develop. The fetus's skin is so transparent that its blood vessels are visible. The fetus now starts to swallow amniotic fluid which it excretes via the bladder. The first feces start to accumulate in the bowels.

you

minor discomforts

Most women enjoy these weeks. They revel in their obvious pregnancy, but are still not too big to be slowed down by it. There are a couple of potential minor problems that some, but by no means all, women suffer from, starting around now.

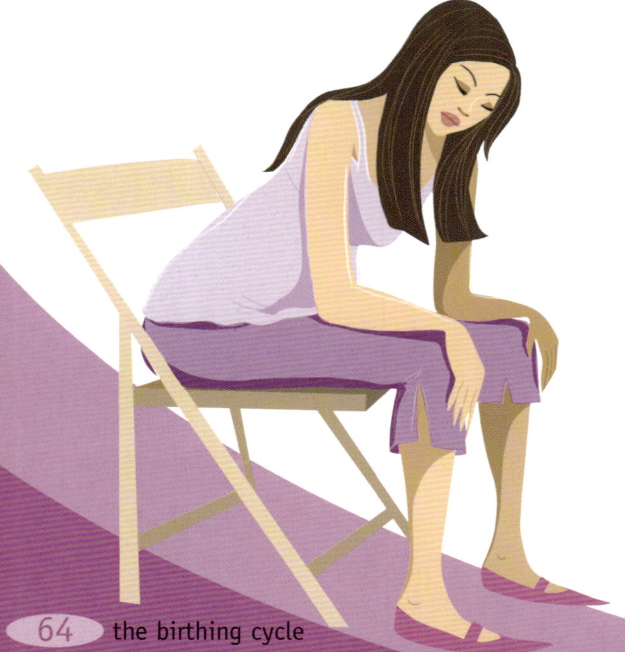

feeling faint?

Changes in the volume and circulation of blood during pregnancy can cause dizziness. If you feel faint, lower your head between your knees. When you rise from a sitting position, do so slowly. If you stand a lot at work, take a walk every so often to help maintain circulation.

hemorrhoids

As the uterus starts to put pressure on your veins, hemorrhoids (swollen blood vessels around the anus) may result. Depending on their severity, you may experience pain or itchiness. There are a number of topical agents you can apply to ease discomfort. Also, try applying an ice pack. Constipation can make things worse, which you can avoid by eating a high-fiber diet and drinking plenty of water.

second trimester

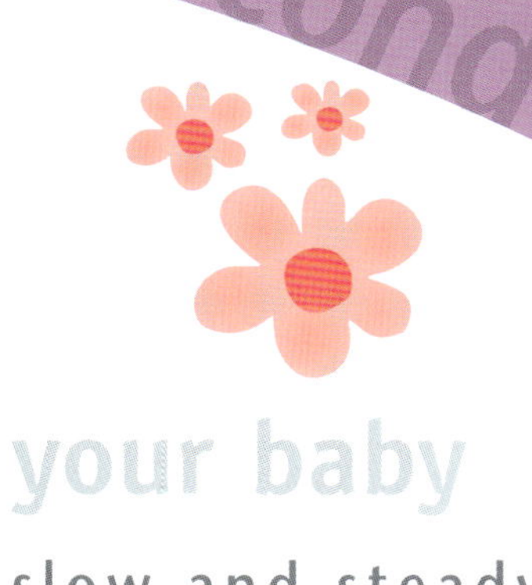

your baby

slow and steady

Many of the same processes continue during these weeks, making your baby bigger and stronger. Muscles get stronger. Legs and arms grow longer. The fetus has finger- and toenails. The first teeth start to harden in the jaw. Tooth tissues give rise to dentine, a harder-than-bone substance that forms the body of teeth, and enamel, the glossy substance found on the surface of teeth. A very few babies are actually born with a tooth; for most, teeth will start to erupt from the gums in the latter months of their first year.

you

stay in shape

If you are taking an exercise class, always tell the instructor that you are pregnant. If necessary, routines and movements can be modified for you.

Following some kind of fitness program during the course of your pregnancy will really pay off when it comes time to give birth. Well-toned muscles can contribute to an easier, less painful labor. If you were exercising regularly before you got pregnant, you should be able to continue with a similar regimen well into your pregnancy. If you are new to regular exercise, be sure to consult your doctor beforehand. Useful guidelines are as follows:

- Try to set aside 10–15 minutes every day for exercise
- Always start with a series of gentle warm-up exercises
- Do not continue with anything that causes pain or fatigue

Try walking, swimming, and cycling (early on). Avoid exercises such as skiing or horse riding.

your baby

fighting infection

The immune system starts to develop, and antibodies—proteins used by the immune system to neutralize bacteria and viruses—can be detected for the first time. Your baby will be born with these natural immunities, and you will transfer many of your immunities to your baby if you breast-feed.

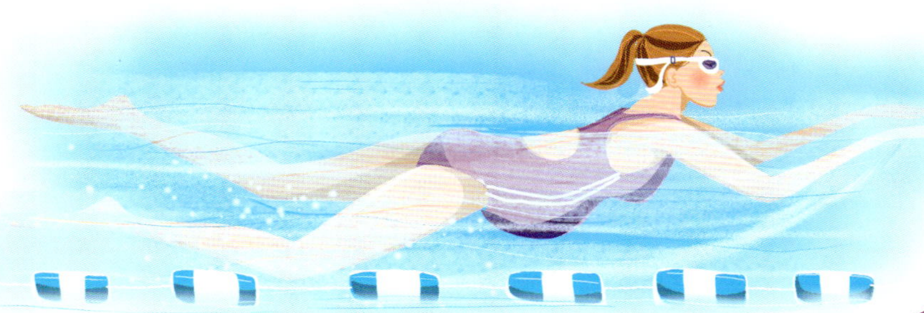

second trimester

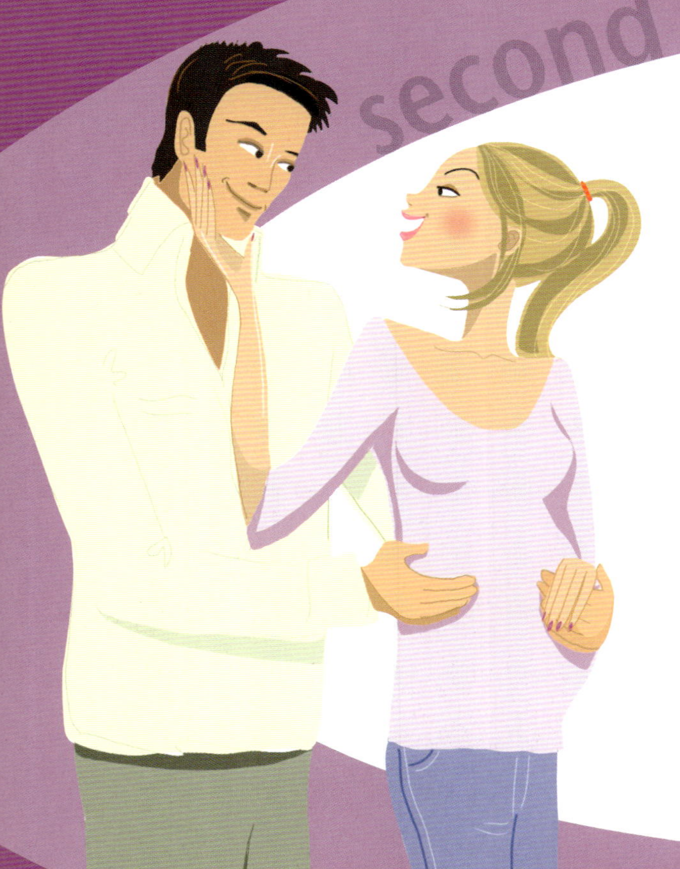

you

pregnancy highs: renewed sex drive

For many women, the second trimester is one of higher energy levels and the return of a healthy sex life. Up until now, the novelty of being pregnant and the nausea and fatigue that come with it were probably enough to put you off sex altogether. Now, however, the increased hormones in your body, together with sensitive breasts and genital area make sex more stimulating than ever. Furthermore, you have no concerns regarding contraception.

your baby

sleeping and waking

Your baby's sleep-wake cycle is established: it is active more than 50 percent of the time and you will often be able to tell these periods apart as your pregnancy advances. When the fetus is awake, it sucks amniotic fluid and excretes it through the bladder in preparation for life outside the womb. It kicks with some regularity, which you will become more aware of as it gets bigger and bigger. It may also suck its thumb and wrinkle its forehead.

For the most part, it is safe to have sex throughout your pregnancy (though check with your healthcare provider if you have any concerns). It can be very positive for your relationship with your partner, as well as beneficial to you physically.

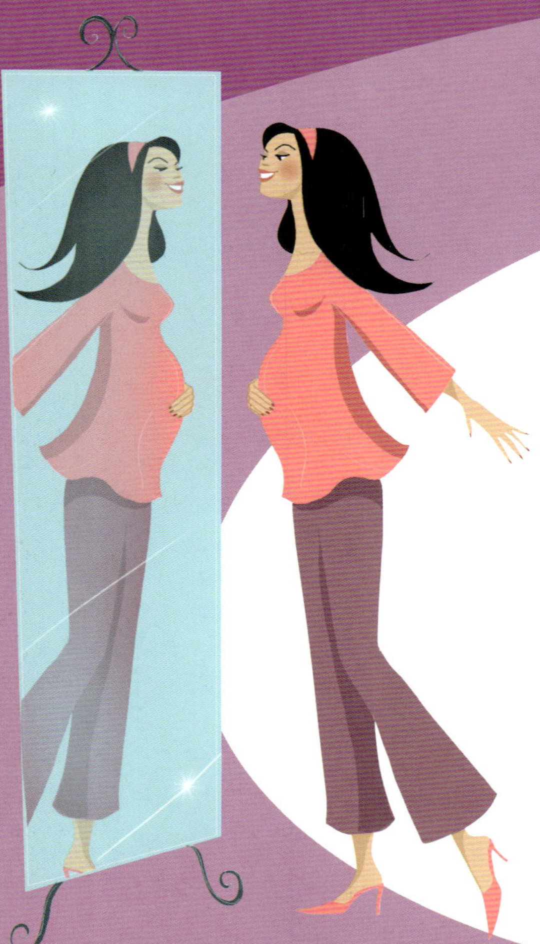

you

looking great

Round about now you should be feeling fabulous. Your bump is not too big, but it won't go unnoticed either. The condition of your skin is considerably improved: dry skin tends to soften while oily skin becomes less so. The increased amount of estrogen in your body works wonders, and your skin is likely to be clear and glowing. However, you are more prone to pigmentation, so protect yourself from strong sunlight. Your hair is likely to become more luxurious as the raised level of hormones causes hair that would normally have fallen out to be retained. This extra hair is then shed after delivery.

your baby

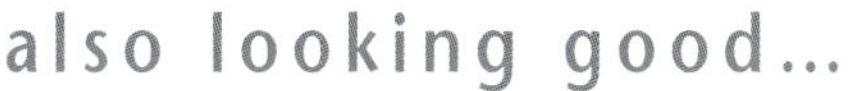

Your baby is getting better looking, too. Lanugo now covers the entire body and there is hair—albeit fuzzy—on the head. The fetus starts to grow eyebrows and eyelashes. Nipples appear. A fatty layer of insulation starts forming around the spinal cord, while brown fat starts accumulating under the skin, making it less transparent.

Your baby starts to manufacture its own kind of moisturizer called *vernix caseosa* (often just called vernix), a protective, white, cheese-like coating made from a mix of oil and skin cells. This coats the skin of the fetus until birth. If your baby is born early, vernix will still be present.

nail facts

Your increased metabolism may make your nails grow faster, which may also cause them to become brittle and to develop grooves. Having a manicure should help, and will improve your feelings of well-being still further.

Your developing baby is approximately 8 inches long and weighs about a pound.

aches and pains

Most pregnancies are largely trouble-free. However, you are unlikely to sail through without some minor problems. Among the most common are varicose veins (which usually become more apparent at around five to six months) and abdominal pain.

pregnancy lows: varicose veins

Increased weight gain, congested blood vessels, and heredity all contribute to varicose (large or swollen) veins. They usually appear in the legs and feet and can be made worse by standing up for long periods of time. Elevating your legs—sleeping with your feet on a cushion, for example—and wearing support hose can help.

pregnancy lows: aches in the lower abdomen

As your uterus grows, the ligaments that support it stretch, which can cause sharp abdominal pain when you stand up after being immobile for a while. The measures on the left should help.

abdominal pain

Try the following self-help measures if you are troubled by abdominal pain:

- Draw your knees up to your chest
- Apply a heating pad
- Bend into the pain

your baby

hello baby

The fetus looks more like a baby every day, with a head that's proportional to the body and long, shapely limbs ending in obvious feet and hands. Unique foot- and fingerprints have now formed and there are creases in the skin of the soles of the feet and the palms of the hands. The hands can make grasping motions, and the baby may suck its thumb. The hair is growing longer and the eyelashes and eyebrows are in place.

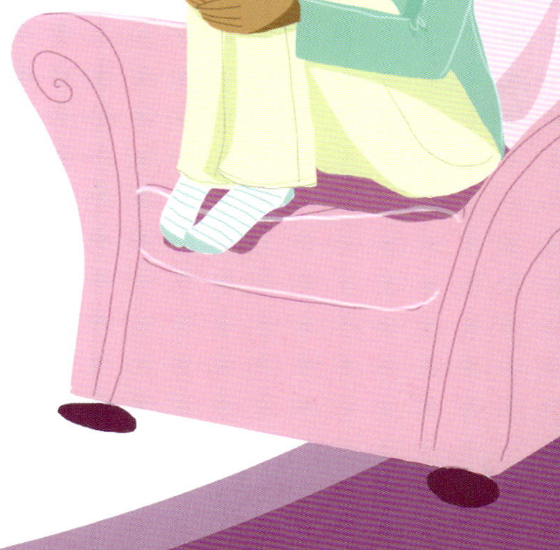

second trimester

you

pregnancy highs: feeling the baby move

Although some women feel their baby move as early as 14 weeks, you are more likely to have to wait until around weeks 18 to 21, particularly if you are a first-time mother. The first fetal movements tend to be felt as a soft fluttering and are in fact just everyday tummy rumblings. As the baby grows, the movements become more distinct, and by about six months they are unmistakable. Your partner will be able to feel the baby move just by resting a hand on your stomach, and you may even be able to tell an arm from a leg as it elbows or kicks from within. Hard kicks can take your breath away, but they are a good sign that your baby is growing healthily.

pregnancy lows: gas, flatulence

Uterine pressure on the intestines, slower bowel movements, eating certain foods, and swallowing air all contribute to gas. Your body needs time to adjust to a high-fiber diet. Make sure you eat small, frequent meals, chew thoroughly, and drink plenty of fluids. Exercise may also be helpful in preventing gas.

your baby

moving around

You will only feel a kick when the baby is facing outward and kicking against your abdominal wall. You won't feel kicks into the uterus.

The fetus is more active than ever. In addition to sucking and kicking, it may respond to unexpected stimulation, such as a sudden touch or sound, with involuntary movements. It may yawn and it may hiccup (which you will feel). It may settle into a favorite position in the womb. Underneath the *vernix caseosa*, the skin is red and wrinkly; there's still not much fat to plump out the skin.

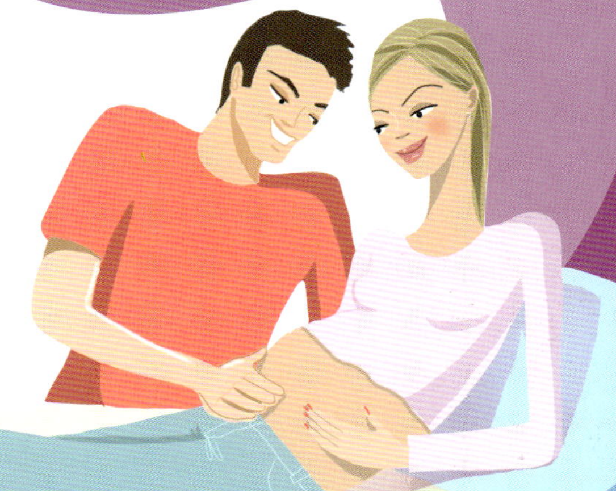

second trimester

you

taking good care of yourself

The following things will help you to adjust to your new looks and feel good about yourself:

- With your doctor's permission, engage in moderate exercise, such as a daily walk (see p. 66)
- Make sure you eat a healthy, balanced diet (see p. 89)
- Get plenty of rest
- Pamper yourself with a new haircut (but avoid coloring your hair)
- Stock up on some colorful scarves or other accessories to dress up your maternity outfits
- Have a manicure or pedicure
- Wear comfortable shoes
- Make positive affirmations to yourself about the physical changes in your appearance—you look great

good shoes

The good news is that the pregnancy hormone relaxin, which relaxes all your muscles in preparation for birth, also relaxes the tissues in the feet, which usually means you will need new shoes—probably a half a size larger. This effect is unlikely to occur in a second pregnancy.

your baby

your baby's senses

By around six months old, the structure of the eyes is complete, and they are now almost ready to open. Tests have shown that at this stage there is a response to light, which is perceived by the fetus as a faint, reddish glow. The fetus can also now hear, and can hear your heartbeat and the sound of your blood pumping around your body. Some mothers-to-be make a point of talking to their unborn babies. You could also play gentle music—evidence suggests that this can make a baby more restful.

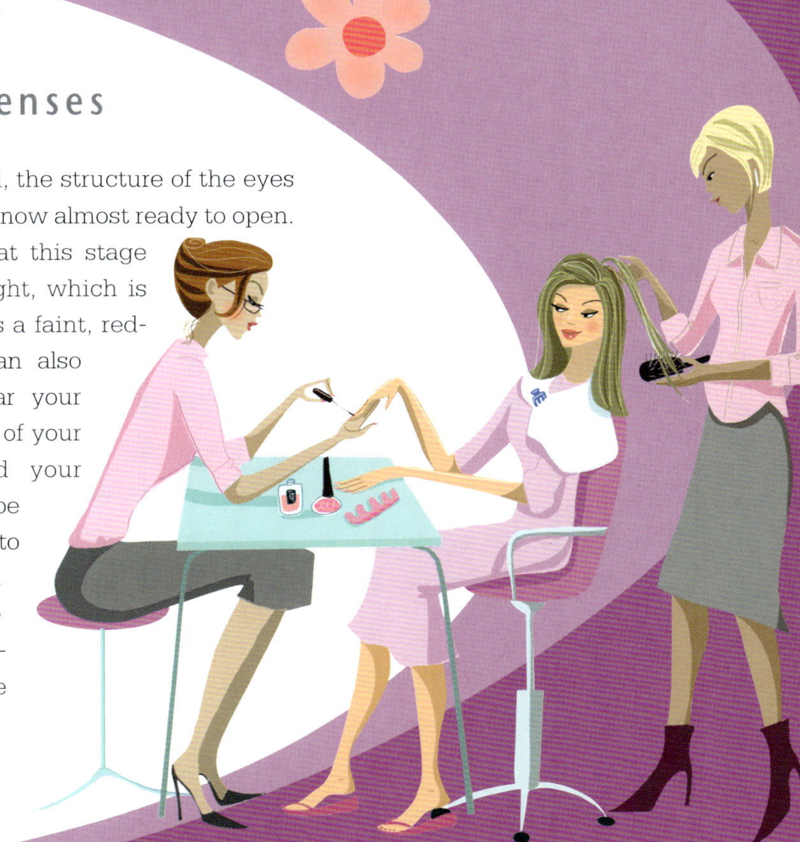

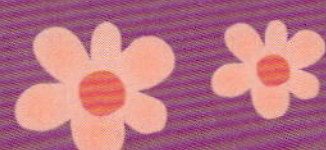

you

a possible health problem: gestational diabetes

Gestational diabetes affects about four percent of all pregnant women.

It is possible to develop gestational diabetes toward the end of your pregnancy, even if you have not had diabetes before. This is because your body is less able to produce all the insulin that is needed to help keep blood sugar levels down. Gestational diabetes can be harmful. It raises your baby's birth weight, which increases your risk of a difficult labor, or delivery by cesarean section (see pp. 120–121). Gestational diabetes can be treated and, in most cases, will involve regular testing of your blood sugar level, eating a healthy diet, and regular exercise. Your doctor may also prescribe insulin as part of a treatment plan.

At six months old, the fetus is around 11 inches from head to heel and weighs slightly more than 1½ pounds.

am I at risk?

You are at risk if:

- You have a history of diabetes in your family
- You have had gestational diabetes in a previous pregnancy
- You are obese
- You are an older mother (over the age of 30)
- You have had a large baby previously (more than 9 pounds)
- You have a history of pregnancy-induced high blood pressure

your baby

it's bad news for baby, too

High levels of glucose in your body are passed to the baby via the placenta. In order to cope with this, the baby produces more insulin than it needs and, because it has more energy than it can use, it stores the excess as fat. Inevitably, this produces a larger baby with low blood sugar levels at birth. This also predisposes it to obesity and diabetes in later life.

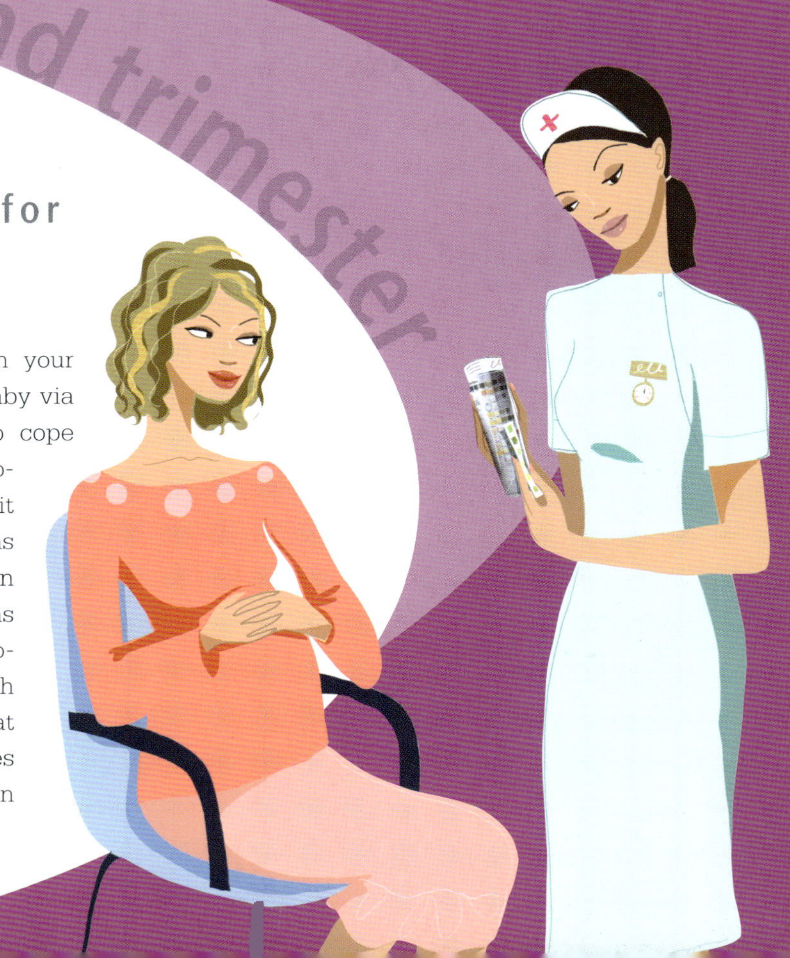

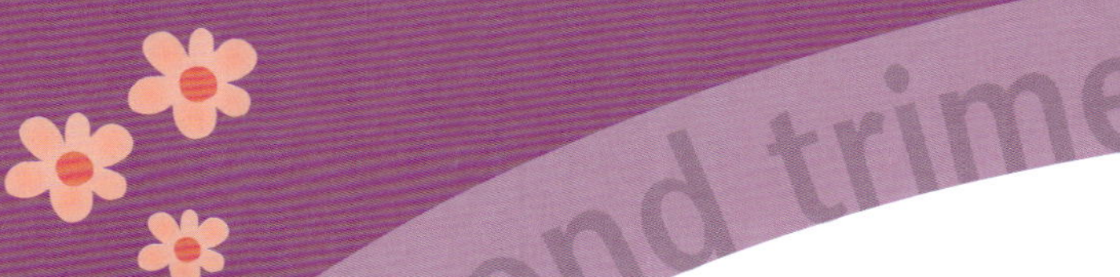

taking a prenatal class

Prenatal classes can be helpful, and are available at most clinics. Classes run over a number of weeks and are given by nurses or other caregivers to a small group of women with similar due dates. Partners are also encouraged to attend. The classes are designed to provide you with a basic overview of pregnancy. Typical topics include fetal development, the benefits of a healthy lifestyle, choosing caregivers, the various birth options, and the pros and cons of breast- and bottle-feeding. In addition to taking part in various discussion groups, you will be encouraged to practice:

- Baby visualization
- Relaxation techniques
- Pelvic floor exercises
- Breathing exercises

questions I want to ask

note down particular concerns about any aspect of labor, birth, and motherhood you wish to address in class use this page to express how you feel after six months; what will you tell your baby about this time?

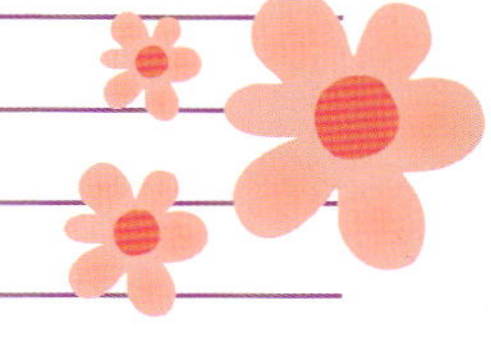

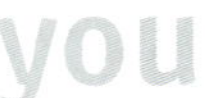

what's happening to me?

You may feel a bit apprehensive as the big day approaches. You may wonder whether you can push the baby out or cope with the pain. Such feelings are common. Childbirth may not be easy, but it is something that women go through successfully every day. Focus on practicing those breathing and relaxation techniques to alleviate some of the anxiety.

how do I feel?

Some of the discomfort you experienced during the first trimester returns, as your internal organs continue to be displaced to make room for your growing baby. You may also feel large and clumsy, all too aware that you require more space to move around in. You might start to waddle. No matter what size or shape you were prior to your pregnancy, you may now long to have your old figure back and fantasize about how great it will be when you are finally able to return to your former self.

your baby

fine tuning

This trimester marks a period of rapid growth for the baby. At six months, it is still very small, but as more body fat is laid down in these months, the fetus will fill out—its weight is likely to increase five-fold between now and the birth. The baby also grows longer—at six months it is likely to be only 60 percent of its length at birth. All the major organs are in place and during these months they mature, so that by the time your baby is born, all its body systems are ready to function properly.

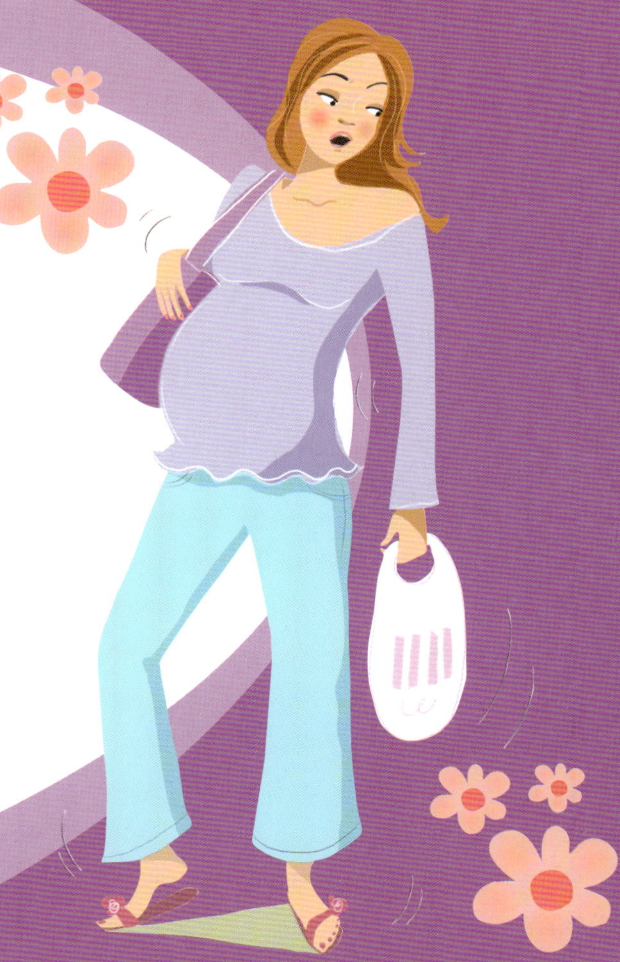

third trimester

you

planning ahead: exploring parenting beliefs

Pregnancy inevitably brings up memories of your own upbringing. Evaluate your childhood and explore any concerns you have about parenting styles with your partner. You may have had a loving childhood and want to emulate your parents' attitudes, or you may have been less fortunate. Either way, discuss parenting together and come up with an approach that fits both of your ideas. Take a look at some of the many books on child development or check out available parenting classes at hospitals and schools: it's never too early to sign up for one. Consistency is important in raising children, and both of you should work toward a unified parenting style.

pregnancy lows: itchy belly

As your abdominal area expands, an increased blood supply to the skin can cause itching. Apply a mild oil, such as almond oil, for comfort. Avoid all aromatherapy oils, because the herbs and stimulants found in some of them might be absorbed through the skin and affect the fetus.

your baby

learning to breathe

The rapidly developing brain and nervous system are now mature enough to take charge of some major functions. The nostrils open. Respiration becomes more rhythmic and is better coordinated. Inside the lungs, minute air sacs called alveoli have formed, and it is now possible for the fetus to "breathe"—that is, to exchange carbon dioxide for oxygen. However, a baby born at this time would need the help of a ventilator for breathing for several weeks.

you

nutrition and weight gain

You need to provide your growing baby with all the right nutrients for its healthy development because your nutritional needs have increased by about 300 calories a day. You can expect to gain somewhere between 25 and 35 pounds if you are of normal weight at the start of pregnancy. Women who are underweight will gain slightly more and those who are overweight should expect to gain less. You'll put on up to 5 pounds during the first trimester and about 1 pound a week thereafter. Make sure you eat balanced (preferably small) meals, spread throughout the day.

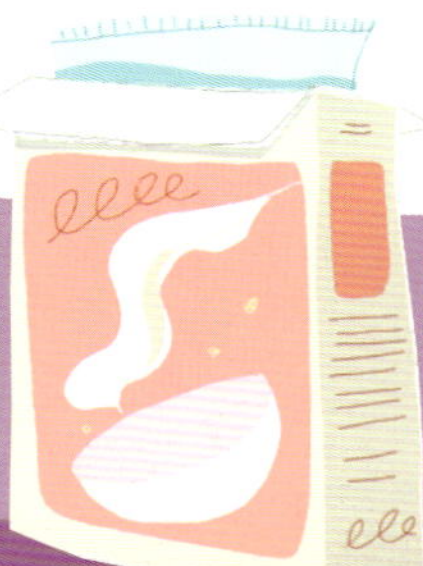

your baby

in touch with the outside world

The fetus reacts more frequently to external sounds. The eyes can open and close reflexively. The fetus may experience rapid eye movements (REM) during sleep. In boys, the testicles descend to the scrotum. Although there is more fat forming under the skin, the fetus is still red, wrinkled, and covered with *vernix caseosa*.

what should I be eating?

- Grains: great for providing energy. Wholemeal varieties are higher in nutrients and are a great source of fiber—essential for keeping constipation at bay (see p. 64)
- Fresh fruit and vegetables: these are essential for providing minerals and vitamins. Eat broccoli, spinach, onions, lima beans, mangoes, raspberries, kiwi fruits, and bell peppers
- Dairy products: high in calcium. Good sources include hard cheeses, natural yogurt, and low-fat milk
- Protein: essential for healthy cell growth and muscle repair. Opt for lower fat sources such as lean chicken breast, firm white fish, beans, and legumes

At the end of week 30, your developing baby weighs between 2½ and 3 pounds and, at almost 14 inches, is two-thirds its final size.

you

nesting instincts

It is not unusual for pregnant women to have a sudden burst of energy during the last trimester, and many find themselves frantically cleaning out kitchen cupboards or scrubbing walls in the nursery just weeks before giving birth. Commonly referred to as the "nesting" instinct, the benefits of such activity are that you feel better about your home, and have more time to spend with your baby once it arrives by reducing the amount of time you need to spend on household chores in the busy first weeks. On the downside, however, you could overdo it and waste precious energy. You are going to need all the resources you can muster once labor starts so go easy on the cleaning and decorating but, if it has to be done, enlist the aid of others.

working and pregnancy

Many women work until well into their pregnancies, preferring to plan to take more time once the baby actually arrives. For most women, this works out well. However, listen to your body. If you are finding that you are very tired or stressed, it might be worth cutting down on your hours or even stopping work altogether sooner rather than later. Discuss your options with your partner, doctor, and of course, your employer.

your baby

arriving early

The fetus's level of infection-fighting antibodies now equals yours. With a good deal of effort and expert intensive care, the fetus might be able to survive outside the womb, but complications are likely. The good news is that about 85 percent of babies born at 28 weeks survive, and this percentage rapidly increases so that a 35-week baby is almost certain to be fine.

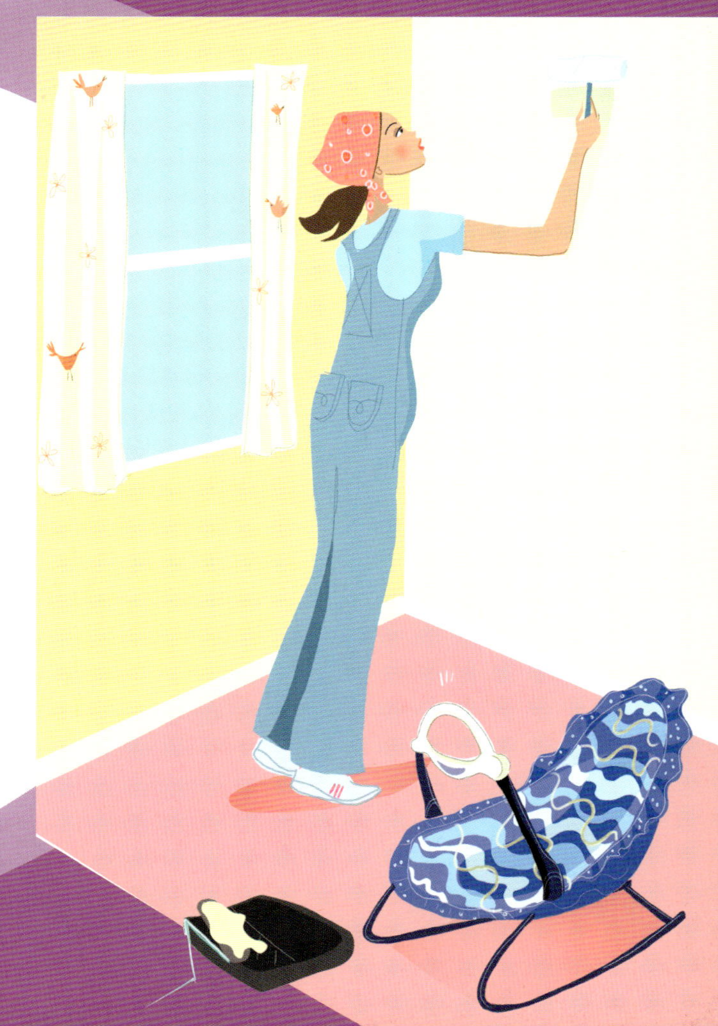

you

minor discomforts

The last few weeks can be a time of minor, niggling discomforts. But keep in mind that your baby is nearly here and that it will all be worth it when you hold him or her in your arms.

leg cramps

You may start to get leg cramps. These are usually caused by a combination of poor circulation, fatigue, compressed nerves, and an imbalance of essential minerals. Avoid pointing your toes, as this can easily bring on cramping. Use warm compresses, massage, and gentle exercises to stretch your leg and foot muscles. One option is to evaluate your diet, and your doctor may suggest that you take a calcium supplement to change the balance of minerals in your system.

breathlessness

In the last trimester, you may find yourself increasingly short of breath as the uterus pushes up, putting pressure on the diaphragm. Beginners are lucky—first-time moms will find relief toward the last few weeks of the pregnancy, as the fetus moves down into position. Women who have given birth before will have to wait until labor starts to get relief.

third trimester

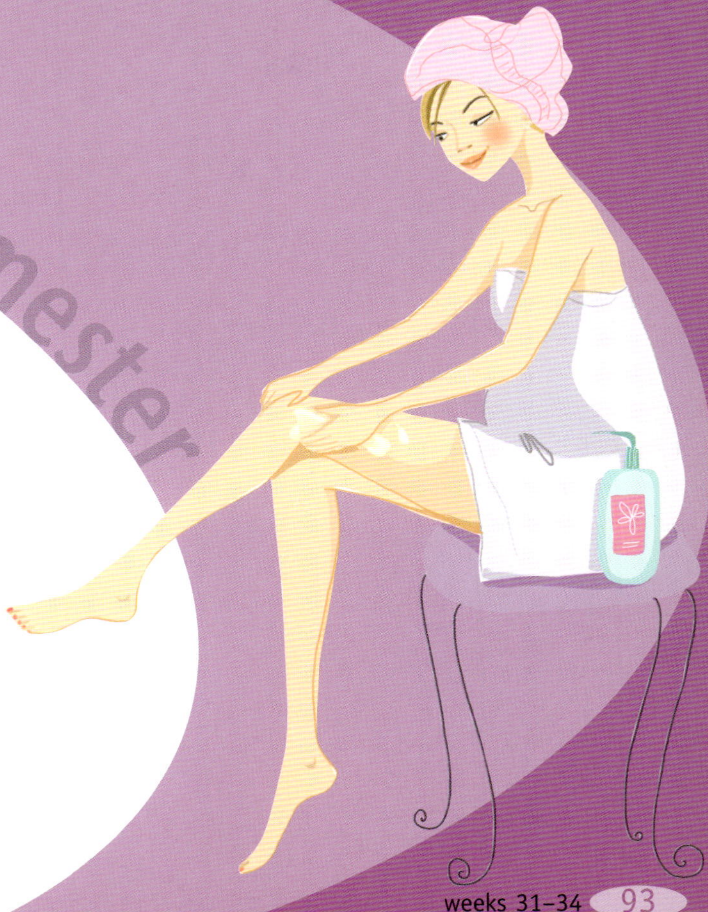

your baby

breathe in, breathe out

The lungs are maturing in readiness for life outside the womb. Your baby is helping in this process, by breathing in amniotic fluid and then expelling it. This is not a constant process, but it does stimulate lung development.

you

what is your partner thinking right now?

Chances are, your partner is anxious. Perhaps he is worried about an increased sense of financial responsibility if you are planning to stay home from work, even for a short while. Or maybe he does not know how to reconcile working longer hours with your expectations that he also help with childcare duties. He may be struggling with sexual feelings—wondering if the newborn will take your attention and love away from him. He may feel pressured to be the one who is in command—even while feeling a bit out of control. On the other hand, in the months since conception, your partner has had plenty of time to adjust psychologically to the idea that you are both in this together, in which case he will be expressing his love for you and concern for the baby in his own, unique way.

Even the most anxious fathers-to-be relax into fatherhood once the baby arrives. Talk together how you see your upcoming roles and reassure each other that you are going to be fine.

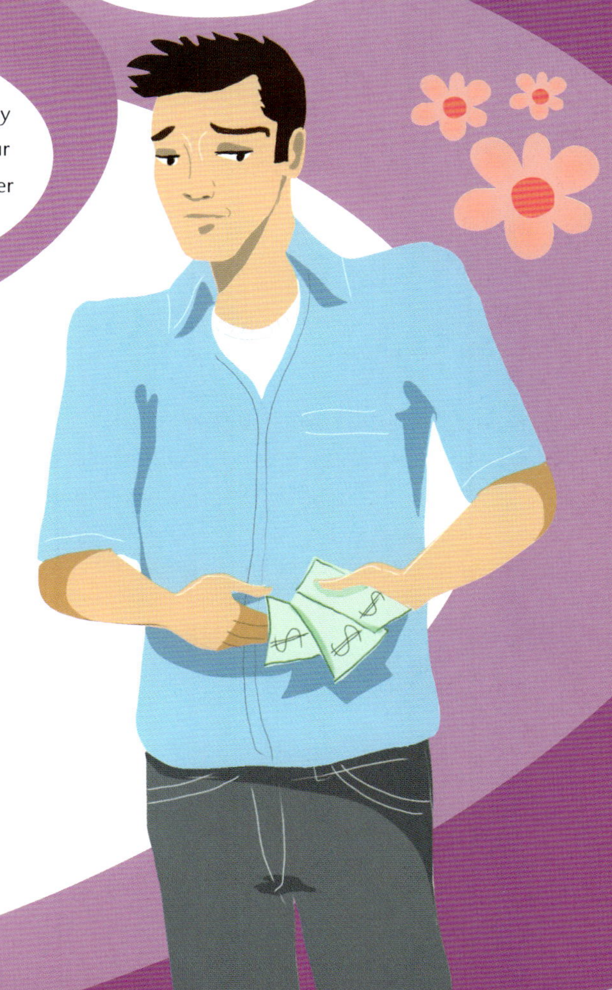

your baby

slowing down

As your baby grows, it becomes more constrained, and doesn't move around as much as it did previously. This quite normal. If it seems as if a long time has elapsed since you last felt movement, have a snack, then lie down and see if your baby reacts by moving. Chances are good that you will feel the baby stir.

third trimester

you

backache

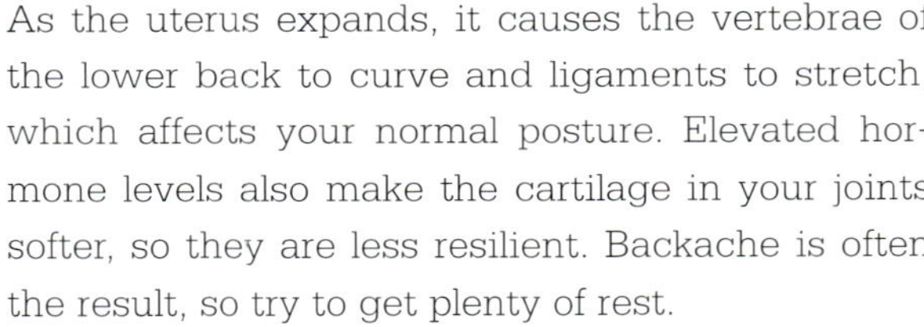

As the uterus expands, it causes the vertebrae of the lower back to curve and ligaments to stretch, which affects your normal posture. Elevated hormone levels also make the cartilage in your joints softer, so they are less resilient. Backache is often the result, so try to get plenty of rest.

backache prevention tips

Ask your doctor about safe exercises to strengthen abdominal and back muscles. Partial sit-ups, done with bent knees and feet flat on the floor, and the pelvic tilt (see left), can help. Also:

- Lift items by bending your legs, not your back. Carry items close to your body
- Place a firm cushion at the small of your back when sitting down
- Swim to reduce back strain from weight gain during pregnancy
- Wear supportive shoes
- When you sleep, lie on your side with a pillow between your knees

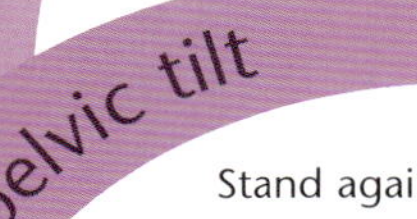

pelvic tilt

Stand against a wall. Press your spine against the wall, tighten your abdominal muscles, and tuck your buttocks down and under your body, so your pelvis tilts upward at the front. You can practice the pelvic tilt in the same way on all fours on the floor.

your baby

eye color

Although your baby's final eye color will not be clear for some months after the birth, around this time, the iris color starts to appear. Most fair babies are born with blue eyes, and most darker-skinned babies with brown eyes, but this may change. The pupils start to dilate, and the post-birth pattern of sleeping with eyes closed, and having them open at other times is established.

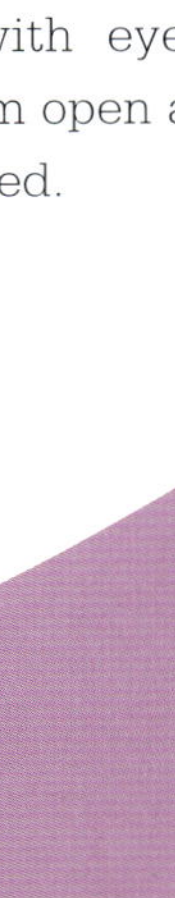

you

how are you sleeping?

Despite being quite tired, you may start to have trouble sleeping through the night. One reason for this is that your sleep patterns begin to mirror those of your baby: the amount of non-REM sleep you get decreases, while your REM sleep increases. This means that you spend less time in deep sleep and are likely to wake more frequently and with greater ease. This is frustrating, but it does seem to serve the purpose of preparing you for the weeks following the birth, when you will need to wake several times during the night to feed and change your baby.

what can I do?

- Try to rest as much as possible during the day
- Don't drink anything for an hour before bedtime and go to the bathroom before turning in
- Take a warm, relaxing bath before you go to bed
- Sleep with a pillow under your belly and/or between your legs
- Avoid sleeping on your back
- Try some visualization and relaxation techniques
- Listen to some calming music
- Get up and make a cup of caffeine-free tea

your baby

moving into position

At some point toward the end of this month, your baby may turn into the final birthing position, usually head down. A small percentage (less than five percent) of babies are "breech," that is, with their legs or bottoms down. Increasingly, doctors advise a cesarean for breech babies as the safest way to deliver the baby and avoid fetal distress.

Your developing baby is gaining weight, thanks to an increase in muscle and fat. It now weighs about 4½ pounds and is between 15 and 17 inches long.

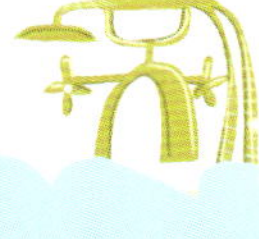

making a birth plan

As you approach full term, your thoughts on how you want to give birth will become clearer. This is the time to write down your preferences by making a birthing plan. There are several issues you may want to consider and these include:

- Who will your birthing partner be? Do you want him/her to be present throughout?
- Have you discussed your birthing options with your caregiver?
- What kind of pain relief do you want (see pp. 116–117)?

medical intervention

- Are you aware that your water may be broken for you if it doesn't break itself? Do you want to avoid an episiotomy? Do you mind the placenta being delivered with the aid of drugs?
- Do you want your baby monitored throughout the birth?
- Do you want to watch the baby come out?
- Will you breast-feed, and would you like instruction?
- How long do you want to stay in the hospital?

The majority of women (50 to 80 percent) have made their infant-feeding decision before the sixth month of pregnancy.

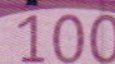

questions I want to ask

note down any questions you wish to discuss with your healthcare provider before finalizing your birth plan

third trimester

you

making room for baby

All expectant mothers really look forward to planning their baby's room, and this is something you and your partner can enjoy doing together. The room should be clean and bright, and there are a number of practical issues you need to think about:

- Wallcoverings should be non-toxic: apply paints or wallpaper glue well in advance so there are no residual fumes
- All electrical outlets should be baby-proofed using covers from the local hardware store
- Make sure the slats in the crib are less than 2⅝ inches apart so the baby's head cannot get caught in between them
- Avoid any dangling strings or cords on the crib or windows: the baby could strangle on them
- Do not place the crib near lamps, electrical appliances, or any other items that could be a safety hazard
- Make sure all linens are secured; do not use pillows in the crib
- Buy nursery toys with contrasting patterns to stimulate interest
- Buy hypoallergenic toiletries and a small bathing tub
- Securely fasten any pad on top of the changing table

your baby

where should the baby sleep?

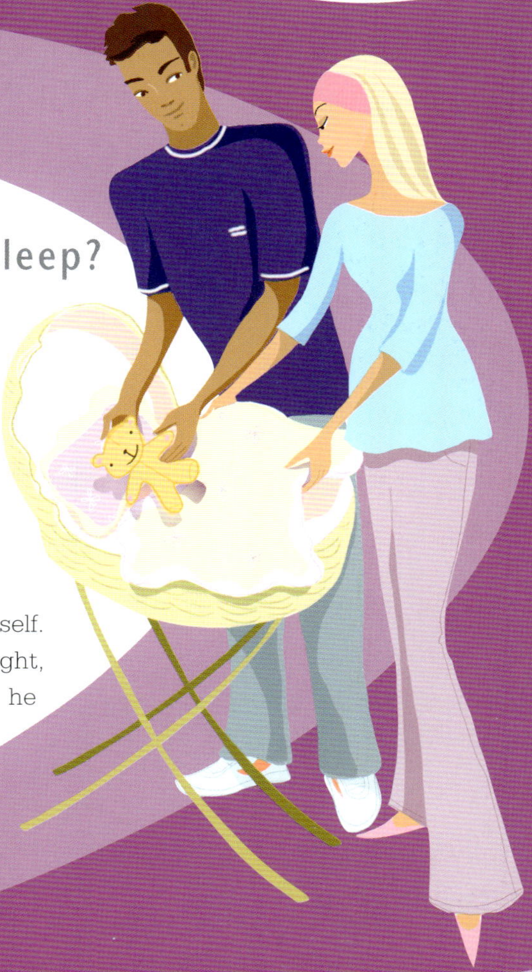

You will want to get your baby's room ready before the birth, as you will have more time then. However, for the first few weeks, most parents choose to have the baby sleep in their room, so that night feedings are easier. If the baby is in a crib at your bedside, you can take him into bed with you, feed him, and settle him back down, and go back to sleep yourself. Once the baby is sleeping through the night, you can move him to the nursery, and he could have his daytime naps there.

you

avoiding stress

As you enter your last month, you are bound to have some anxieties about the birth and your ability to cope as a new mother. Other worries may concern changes in your relationship or that you are unprepared for forthcoming events. Most days, you might be able to cope with the various ups and downs, while others you might find things building up beyond your control. Try the self-help measure here, but if you find it is all getting too much for you, talk to your healthcare provider, as constant stress is not good for the baby.

self-help for stress

Ease stress through relaxation. One very effective method is to lie still with your eyes closed and to relax each of your muscles in turn from head to toe, releasing tension as you go. Breathe slowly and rid your mind of any conscious thoughts.

third trimester

your baby

rounding it out

Over the past few weeks, your baby has been gaining fat, with the result that it is now plumper and the skin is less wrinkled. A good layer of body fat is believed to help in regulating the baby's body temperature in the early days after the birth.

you

prepare yourself

The more you prepare for childbirth, the better off you'll be. Trusted friends and family are always a good source of information about pregnancy, childbirth, and raising children. Their real-life experiences can provide valuable insights and reassurance. Also, visit the birth facility and review any concerns with your healthcare providers. Warn your friends and family members that you will need their help. On the physical side, practice your breathing techniques and work on your abdominals using the exercises taught in your childbirth class.

sibling preparation

If you already have children, you will need to help them adjust to the idea of having a new baby around. Some hospitals run sibling preparation classes. Children gain a realistic sense of what will happen when the baby is born, and parents are shown how to help children adjust.

pregnancy lows: edema

Fluid levels increase during pregnancy, enabling you to keep both your and your baby's body systems running efficiently. Toward the end of your pregnancy, you will find some of this fluid collecting in the lower half of your body, causing your ankles and feet to swell—a condition known as edema. Sitting or standing in one position for long periods of time adds to the problem, so try to have your feet elevated whenever possible and wriggle, rotate, or flex them periodically.

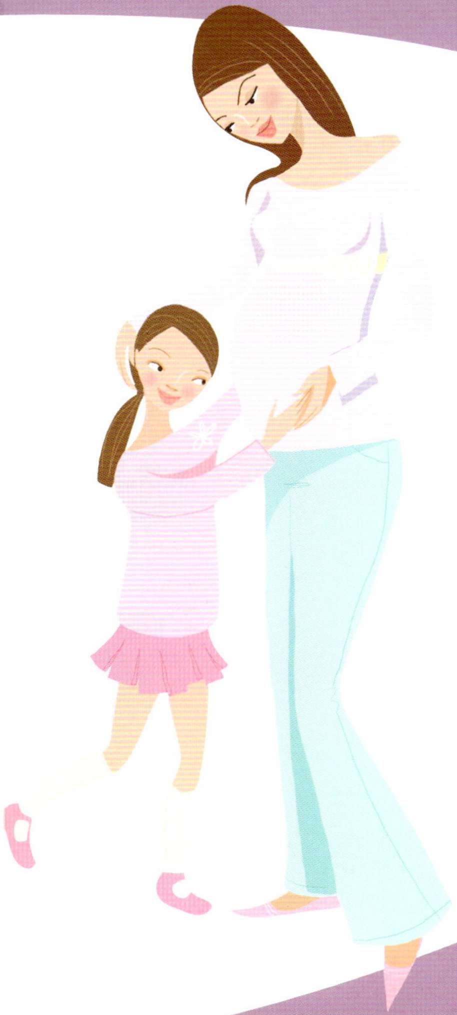

third trimester

your baby

almost there

The lungs are almost fully mature and all the other body systems are almost there, too—a baby born after this time is almost certain to be fine. And many of the "details" are in place: there is likely to be hair on the head, the lanugo and vernix are disappearing (although some may remain in skin folds), the finger- and toenails are fully formed, and the earlobes are in place.

how do I tell false labor from true labor?

Your contractions are getting stronger and more painful. You rush to the hospital but your care provider informs you that it was a false labor. So how can you tell?

signs of false labor:

- Contractions are at irregular intervals
- There is no change in the length or pain of the contractions
- Pain is primarily located in the abdomen
- Walking makes you feel better
- Lying down on your side makes the pain stop

signs of true labor

- Contractions come at regular intervals and increase in length and duration
- Pain moves from back to front
- Walking has no effect on the pain or makes you feel worse
- Contractions continue if you lie down on your side

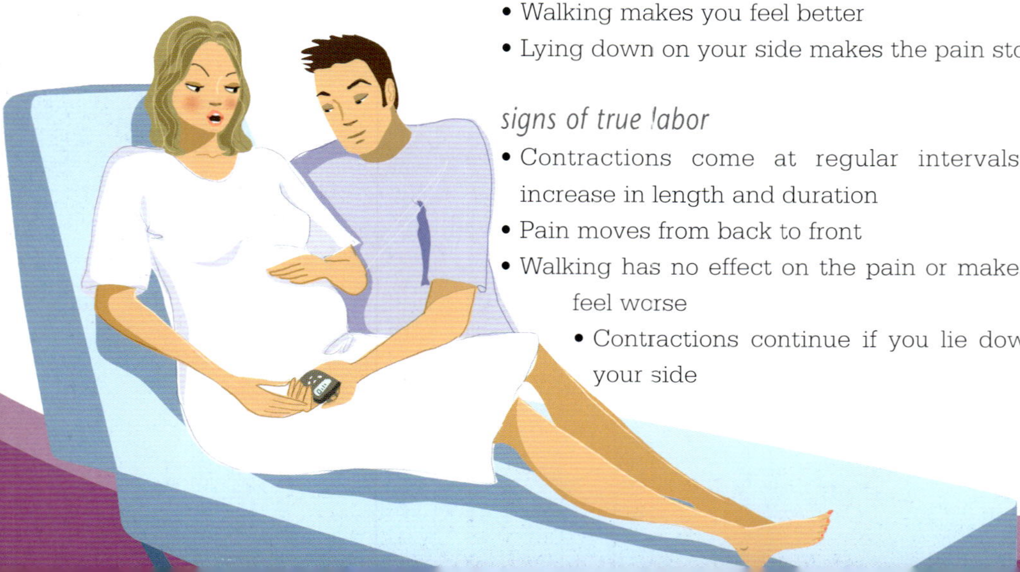

your baby

close to term

Around this point, your baby stops growing and there should be no problems if it is born at any time from now on. The lungs are maturing, a process which will continue after the birth. Because the space in the uterus is now so restricted, your baby cannot move much, so you are unlikely to feel as many kicks and elbows.

warning signs

Not all pregnancies progress smoothly. Below is a list of symptoms that can indicate a serious problem. If you experience any of them, contact your doctor immediately.

Abdominal pain • Bleeding or fluid gushing from the vagina • Blurred vision • Chills • Convulsions • Dizziness • Lack of fetal movement • Extreme headache • High temperature (above 101°F) • Inability to urinate or painful urination • Swollen face and limbs • Vomiting continuously

By 36 weeks, your developing baby weighs between 5 and 7 pounds and is between 16 and 19 inches long.

third trimester

you

what to take to the hospital

Make sure your bag for the hospital is packed at least three weeks ahead of your due date, and be prepared for at least one overnight stay, particularly if this is your first baby.

things for me

- Robe and nightgown
- Slippers with a rubber sole
- Toiletries (toothbrush and paste, hairbrush, deodorant, maxipads, nursing pads)
- Nursing bra and nipple cream
- Change of clothing (with at least two pairs of panties)

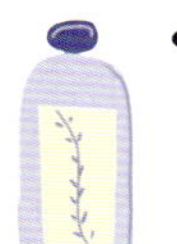

labor aids

- Light snacks and drinks for you and your husband
- Hot water bottle to ease back pain
- Extra pillows for greater comfort

things for baby

- Diapers (although these are sometimes provided by the hospital and charged to your bill)
- 2–3 T-shirts with built-in mittens
- 2–3 sleepsuits
- A blanket
- Going-home outfit, including a hat
- Baby car seat to take baby home in

my list of things to pack

write your own list here and check off items as you put them in your bag

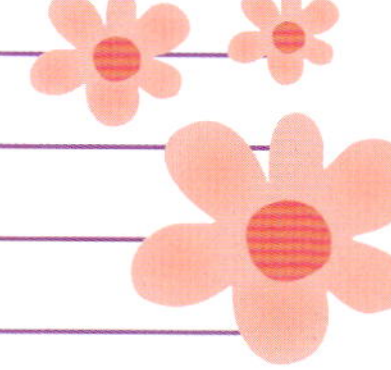

my thoughts and feelings as I get ready to give birth

use this page to sum up how you feel at the end of your pregnancy; what will you tell your baby about this time?

questions I want to ask at the hospital

note down any last questions to ask so that you go into the labor room fully prepared

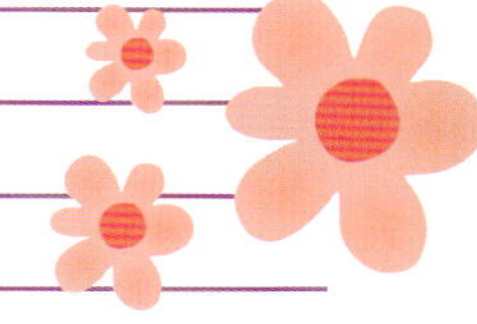

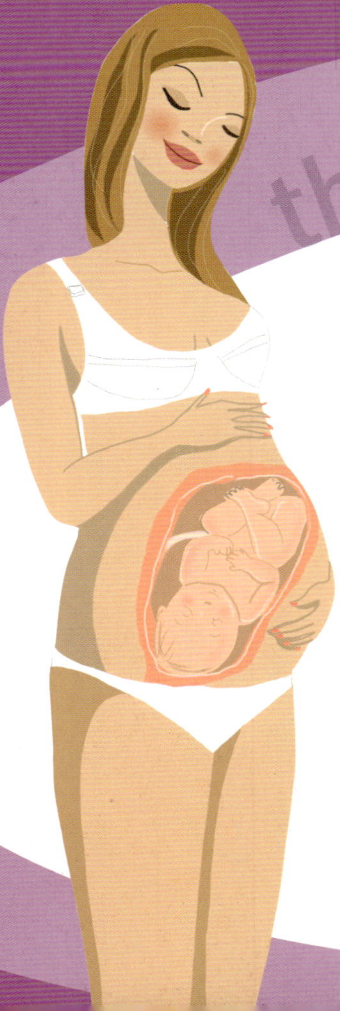

third trimester

you

hormonal changes

As week 40 approaches, the balance of hormones shifts as your body prepares for the birth. Estrogen levels rise, causing the muscles in the walls of the uterus to become more sensitive to oxytocin, the hormone that stimulates uterine contractions. Levels of prostaglandin, a hormone-like substance that stimulates contractions, also rise just before labor.

Your due baby weighs between 7 and 7½ pounds. Most full-term babies are between 18 and 21 inches long.

your baby

into position

The fetus is now considered full-term. Its skin is plump and resilient. The lungs are mature. The mammary glands and external genital structures are visible. There's still some lanugo on the shoulders and back. Some of the *vernix caseosa* remains in folds of your baby's skin, especially around the groin and armpits. There are creases on the soles of the feet. The baby now fills most of the uterine cavity. It moves into the birth position. The head usually points down toward the birth canal, while the arms and legs are pulled close to the chest. Your baby's body rhythms, responses, and activity patterns are well established. Like a newborn, the fetus spends most of the time asleep.

choosing options in pain relief

Every woman's experience of childbirth is different and labor pains vary in intensity from woman to woman. Some feel intense pain throughout the delivery process, while others find the pain less severe. Rhythmic breathing will make the pain created by contractions more tolerable. If a woman's pain becomes severe enough to affect her ability to cope with the repetitive nature of contractions and the length of their duration, then pain relief may be necessary. These are some common options that you should consider before you go into labor:

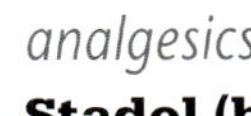

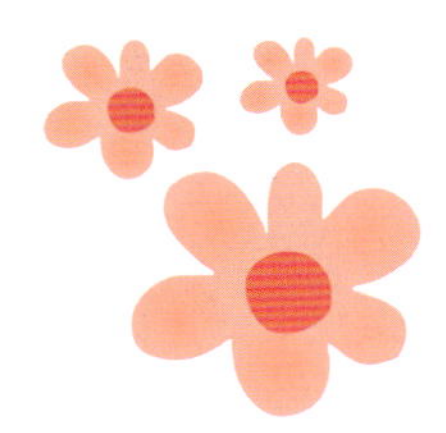

analgesics

Stadol (butorphanol) and Nubain (nalbuphine): these are two common analgesics that relieve pain within minutes but don't eliminate it altogether. This means that they do not cause a complete loss of sensation and so do not inhibit a woman's ability to push during labor. Analgesics are typically given in small doses during the early stages of labor. However, like all drugs, they can cross the placenta and a baby born shortly after a dose of Stadol or Nubain may exhibit respiratory depression. Therefore, these drugs are usually withheld once you reach 2½ inches of dilation. Naloxone (Narcan) may be given to the baby to reverse the side-effects.

anesthesia

Epidural: a regional anesthetic administered by an anesthetist into the "epidural" space of the spinal cord in the lower back. In most cases, it allows women to experience the pressure of the baby moving through the birth canal. Mothers are alert and relatively comfortable throughout delivery. Only small amounts of the anesthetic cross the placenta into the baby because the medications are injected into the epidural space, where they directly block the nerves, rather than into the bloodstream.

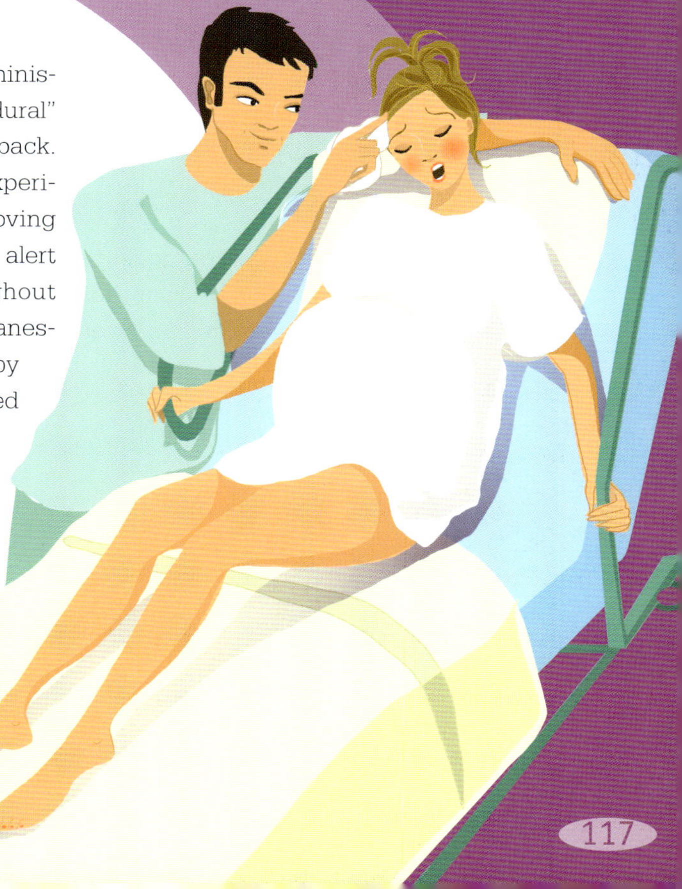

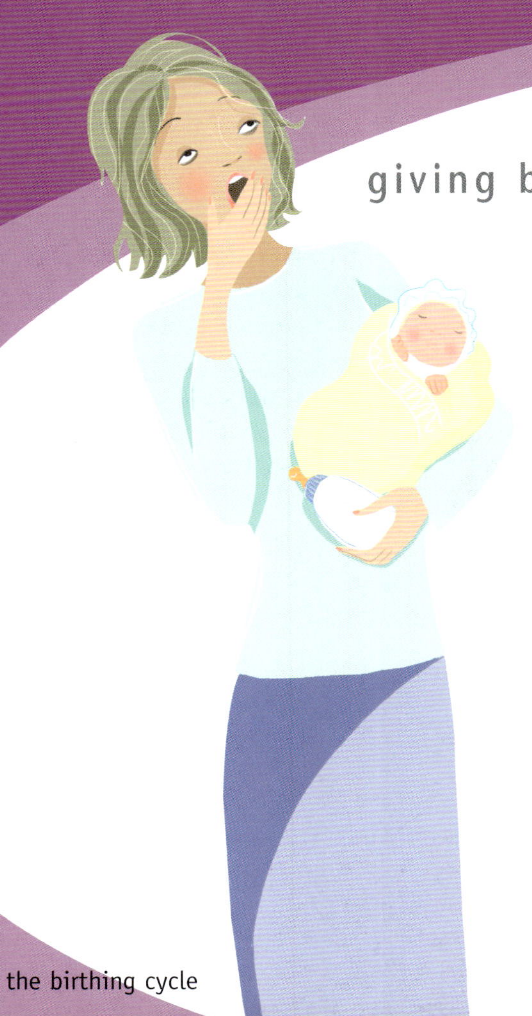

you

giving birth: what to expect

Contractions mark the onset of labor and may occur every 20 minutes and last for about 15 seconds. As labor progresses, the contractions last longer and the time between them shortens, until they occur every two minutes and last for around a minute.

The cervix starts to efface, or thin, and the mucus plugging the opening of the cervix is expelled. With each contraction, the uterus lengthens and narrows, pushing the baby down toward the cervix. The amniotic bag ruptures. The cervix retracts and dilates until it is around 4 inches wide.

The mother pushes with her abdominal muscles, and the

factors for a successful birth

How your baby makes its way into the outside world, and how easy the process will be for you, depends primarily on:

- The shape and size of your pelvis
- The baby's position: most babies come out head first. Birth is more difficult with the feet first (breech)
- The diameter of the baby's head: the head is designed to adjust and usually compresses enough to pass through the pelvis
- Contractions and muscles: during labor, involuntary uterine contractions, together with the mother's use of her abdominal muscles, push the baby out

combination of contractions and pushes causes the vaginal opening to widen and the baby to rotate until it is in position to pass out. Eventually, the baby's head "crowns," or becomes visible. Once the head is through, the body follows easily.

The baby's nose and mouth are suctioned and its umbilical cord is clamped and cut. The baby is placed on the mother, and the mother-infant bonding process begins.

The uterus continues to contract. The placenta detaches from the uterus wall and is expelled 5 to 20 minutes after the birth.

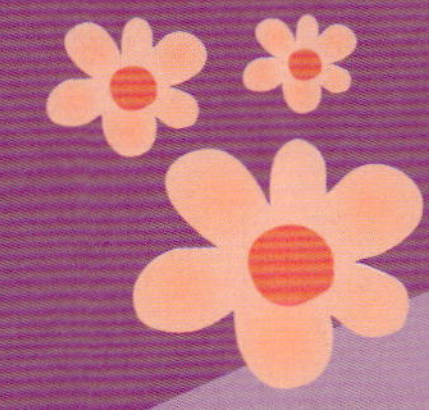

having a cesarean

Complications in the weeks before your due date—or during the birth itself—indicate the necessity for delivery by cesarean section. This is a straightforward procedure, taking 5 to 10 minutes to deliver the baby (and another 30 minutes to complete). It is usually performed under an regional anesthetic such as an epidural, unless there is an emergency, in which case a general anesthetic is given because it acts much faster.

In a non-emergency procedure, the epidural anesthesia is administered into the mother's lower back (meaning she remains conscious throughout). A catheter is inserted to drain the bladder of urine. A small, horizontal incision is made at the base of the abdomen and the amniotic fluid is drained off. The baby is then lifted out, cleaned up, and, if all is well, given to the mother or her partner to hold. The placenta and membranes are delivered last and the incision is stitched up. Doctors leave the intravenous drip and catheter in place for several hours, and remove the stitches a few days later.

common reasons for a c-section

- A forceps delivery fails
- The cervix fails to dilate
- The fetus displays signs of extreme stress
- The baby is in the breech position (feet or bottom first)
- You had a cesarean with a previous baby
- The baby is very large

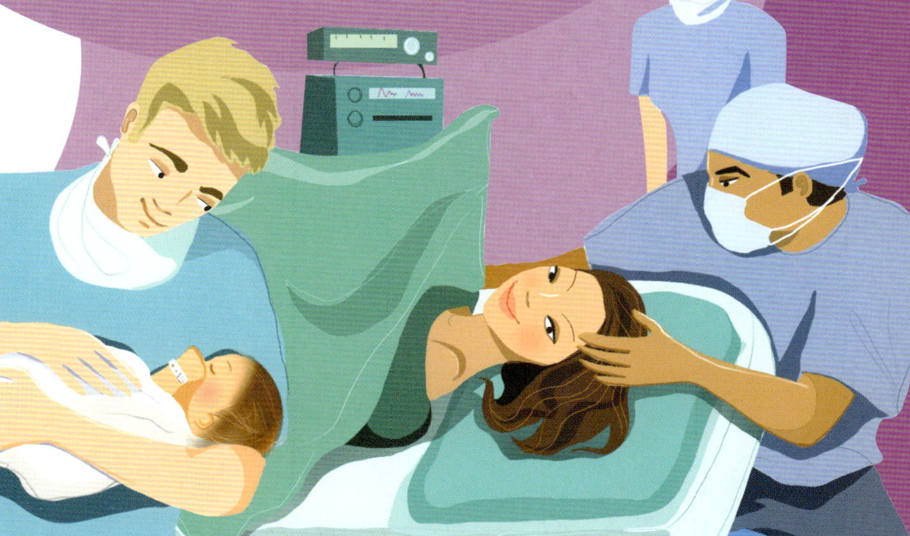

3 the first days and weeks

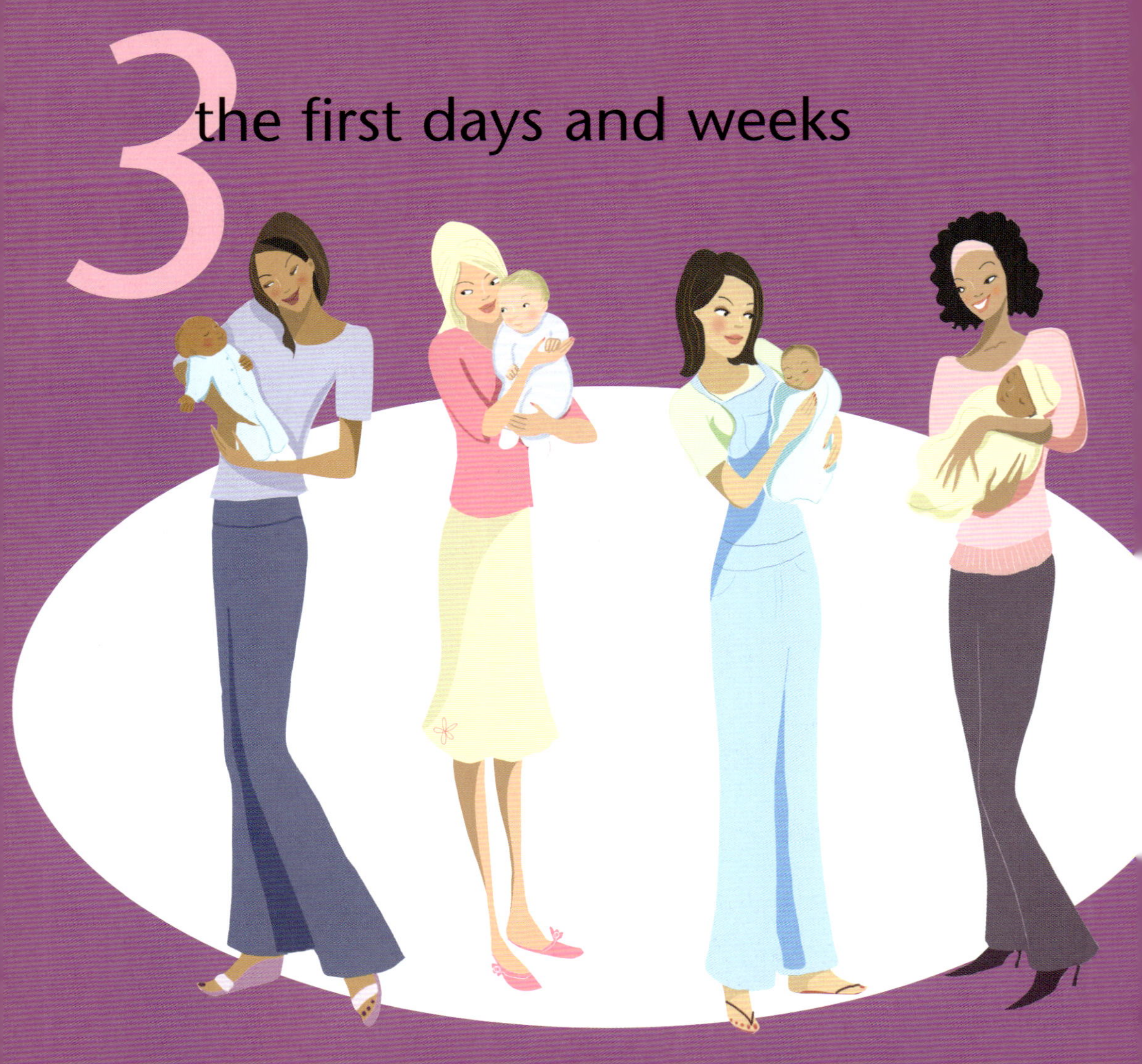

The moment you have been waiting for has finally come—you have delivered a beautiful, healthy baby. What follows is a time of great excitement. Is it a boy or a girl? Who does he look like? How much does she weigh? Despite the efforts of labor for you and your partner, you will both be on a natural high. That is, until the reality kicks in that you are now responsible for this tiny, helpless creature, and have no idea where to start. It is quite normal for you to have anxieties, and for your relationship to take on a new dimension. Take one step at a time, help each other to cope, and once you get to know your baby, you will find it difficult to imagine life without him.

help!

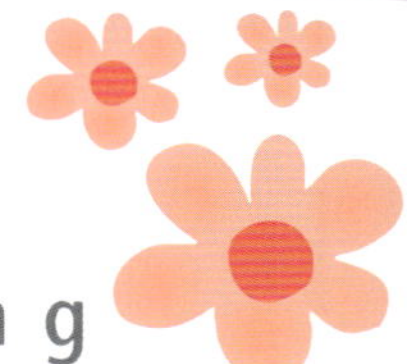

breast-feeding

Breast-feeding is the natural choice for a mother who wants to give her baby the best start in life. You have nurtured her for the last nine months and there is no reason to stop now. At first, your breasts produce a yellowish substance called colostrum. This contains all the necessary nutrients for a perfect feed and provides your baby with the antibodies she needs to fight disease now that she has left the protection of your womb. Colostrum is usually replaced by milk some three days after delivery, by which time you should be well on the way to establishing a feeding routine that works for you and your baby.

baby highs: the pros of breast-feeding

Immediate contact with your baby is your first chance to bond—to see and touch each other for the first time and to establish your role as provider and protector. A newborn baby who has early contact with its mother is quicker to latch on properly than a baby who is separated from its mother in the hour or two following birth. Breast-feeding is convenient. No matter where you are, food is instantly available with no need for sterilization or preparation.

The stimulation of nipples during breast-feeding triggers the release of oxytocin, which makes the uterus contract and reduces the risk of heavy postpartum bleeding.

help!

bottle-feeding

If you choose to bottle-feed your baby, then your feedings will be every three or four hours after delivery. The huge benefit here is that your partner can do it, too, which means he gets to play an active and personal role in the raising of your baby right from day one. You need to sterilize any equipment you use and to prepare fresh formula for each feed. You can hold the baby in much the same way as you would for breast-feeding: semi-upright and supporting the head. To make sure the baby does not swallow air during a feed, tip the bottle up until the formula fills the neck.

baby lows: swallowed air

A bottle-fed baby swallows air more easily during feeds than a breast-fed baby does. This can make him uncomfortable and agitated, so you should burp him every so often. You have three options:

1. Place him over your shoulder and gently pat or rub his back.
2. Sit him upright, lean his weight forward against the heel of your hand, and gently pat or rub his back.
3. Place him facing down on your lap and rub or pat his back.

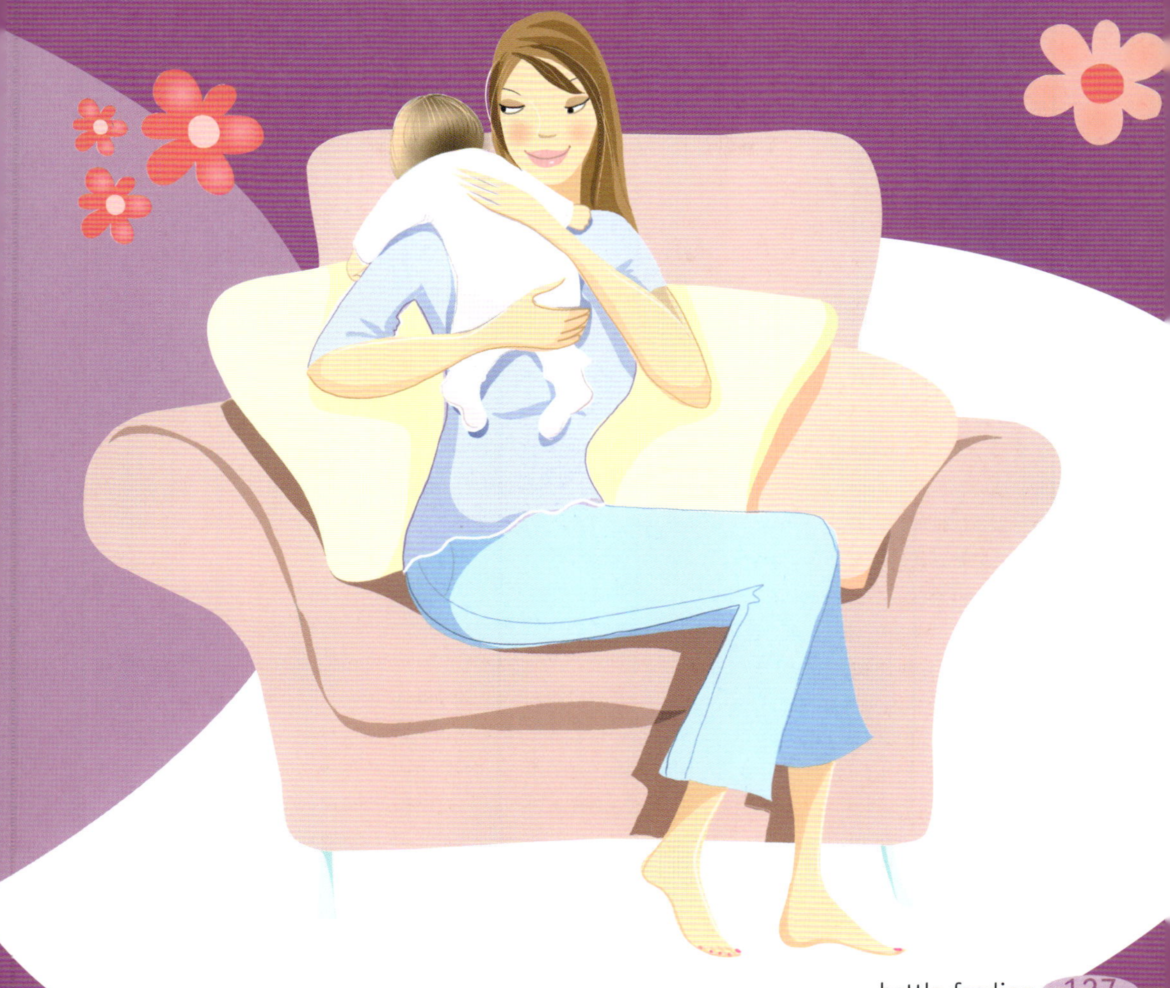

help!

feeding, sleeping, crying

For the first week or two, at least, you and your partner will feel as if you are working around the clock to provide and care for your new baby. No sooner has she had a feeding than she needs bathing; no sooner has she had a nap than she needs changing. The cycle is repetitive and exhausting and the sooner you can settle into a routine that works for you, the more normal your days will become.

what to expect

Feeding: bottle-fed babies tend to settle into a routine quicker than breast-fed babies, feeding every three or four hours. Breast-fed babies are more likely to be fed on demand in the early days, which could mean as few as two hours between feeds. During the night, your baby will wake up at least twice for a feeding.

Sleeping: in the beginning, your baby will sleep for most of the time between feedings, waking only if she is too hot, too cold, or hungry. She will establish more of a routine as time passes and it is important for you to establish a difference between night and day routines early on.

Crying: your baby gets your attention in the first weeks by crying. It may seem that she cries all the time, but you will soon be able to tell whether she is hungry, tired, lonely, or uncomfortable.

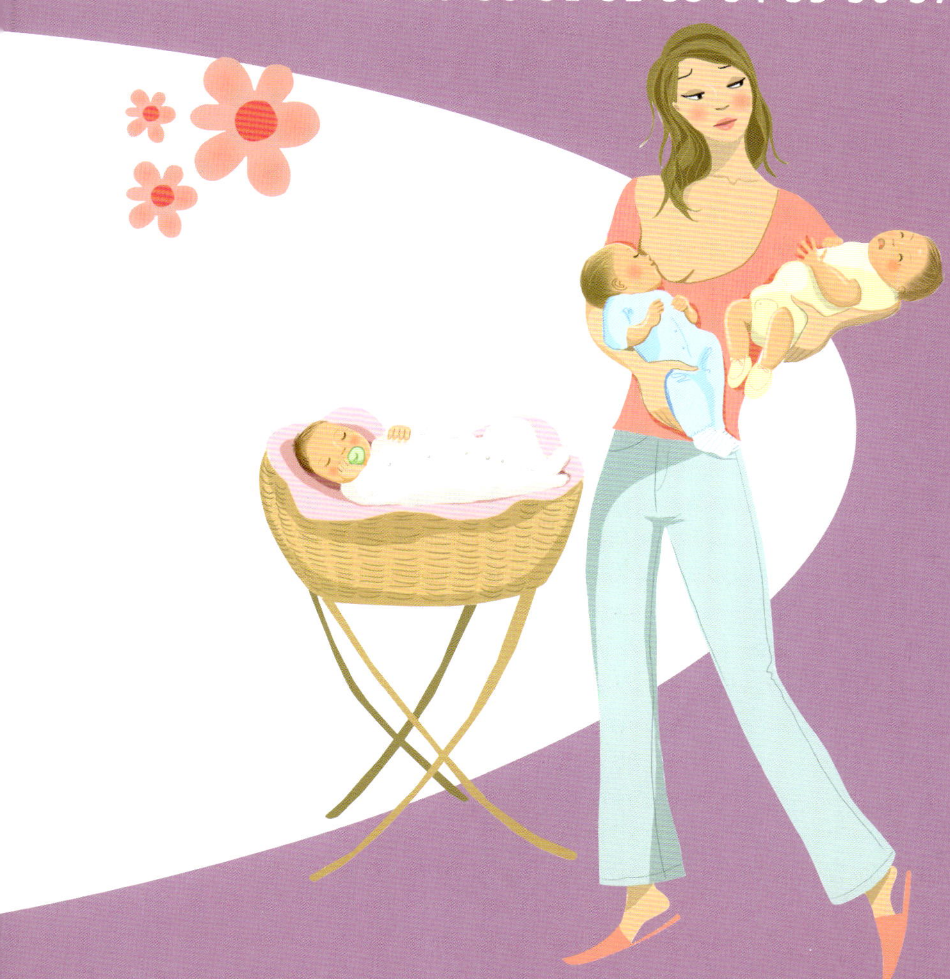

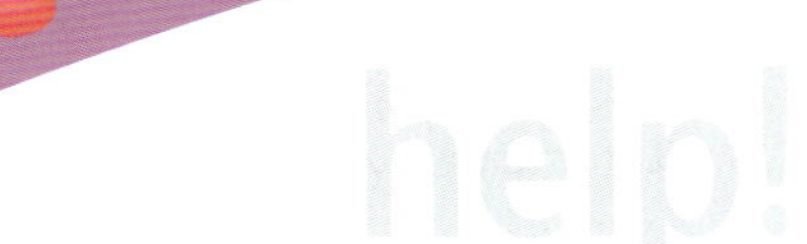

help!

changes to your body

Depending on the nature of your labor, expect your body to feel the effects of delivery for at least a few weeks. You will want to recover any energy lost and should try to rest as often as possible in the first few days. You are also likely to be disappointed with the rather saggy stomach you now have. Expect your body to change in other ways, too.

likely developments

Abdominal pain: you may experience afterpains immediately following the birth, as your uterus begins to contract to its pre-pregnant size.

Lightheadedness: it is normal to feel dizzy in the first few days, while your cardiovascular system adjusts to a reduced volume of blood in circulation.

Bleeding and vaginal discharge: the uterus continues to discharge leftover blood and tissue, called lochia, for a few weeks.

Leaking urine: you may suffer "stress incontinence" while your bladder and pelvic organs return to their pre-pregnancy positions.

Profuse sweating: you will sweat more during the first few weeks as your body gets rid of the excess fluids accumulated during pregnancy.

Engorged breasts: the breasts swell and harden as they begin to produce milk for your baby, and this may be painful. You can massage your breasts to ease the problem. Once the baby learns to nurse properly and your feedings become regular, your breasts should feel less full.

help!

the baby blues

For 10 to 20 percent of new moms, the baby blues develop into "postpartum depression" that, if left untreated, will become worse and last for a longer time, so get help as soon as possible.

It is not uncommon to feel weepy a couple days after the birth. Not only are you tired from the efforts of labor, but your body is going through a new round of hormonal changes, possibly causing you to feel tearful, moody, anxious, and depressed. In most situations, the feelings pass within a few days. If they do not, and you feel your depression getting out of control, you should seek medical advice without delay.

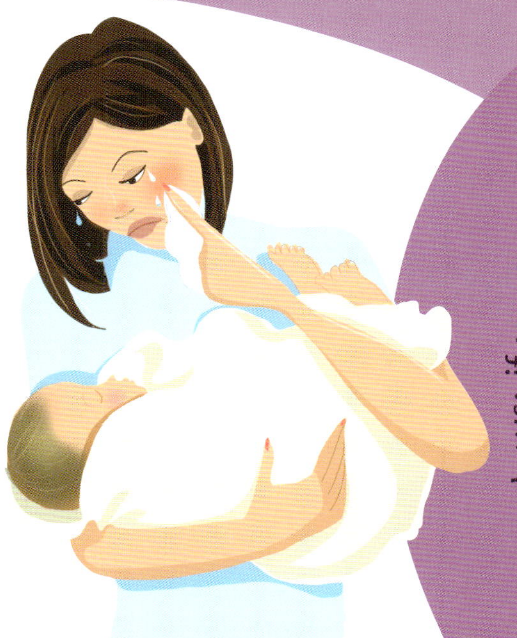

baby lows: if you're feeling blue

After the thrill of seeing your baby for the first time, you may start to feel a sense of anticlimax. Below are feelings that some mothers experience at what is an exciting time, but also a time of great change. You may start to worry about whether you're going to be a great mom as you try to cope with the many demands of your new baby. You may even feel resentful that your life has now completely changed. Giving birth is exhausting, and like all exhausted people, you may feel easily irritated or indecisive. Developing a bond with your baby may also take longer than you think, and this can be frustrating or even distressing.

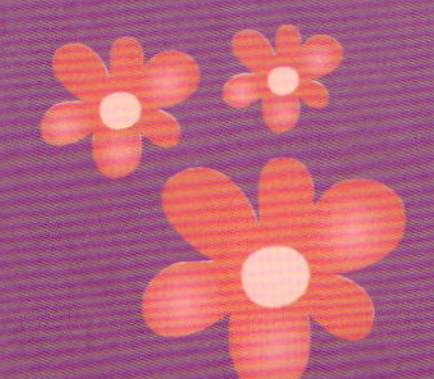

help!

your partner's feelings

The arrival of your new baby will be a life-changing experience for both you and your partner. Although he is close to the action, however, it is impossible for him to feel the same way toward the baby as you do. You carried and nurtured the growing fetus and now feel a tremendous sense of attachment to the baby as well as a strong desire to protect her. The baby must be the center of your attention early on, and your partner may well develop feelings of jealousy. Encourage him to express his feelings and concerns and find ways of involving him in the day-to-day: the sooner he gets used to having the baby around, and to handling and holding her, the more confident he will become in his new role as Dad.

- If you are bottle-feeding the baby, let your partner carry out one or two feedings a day
- Let your partner change and dress the baby frequently, and actively encourage him to do so

- Make bath time a family time, with both of you washing and playing with the baby
- Always find time to be alone with your partner, if only for half an hour a day. This will give you valuable time together
- Make sure your partner and the baby get to spend precious time alone together

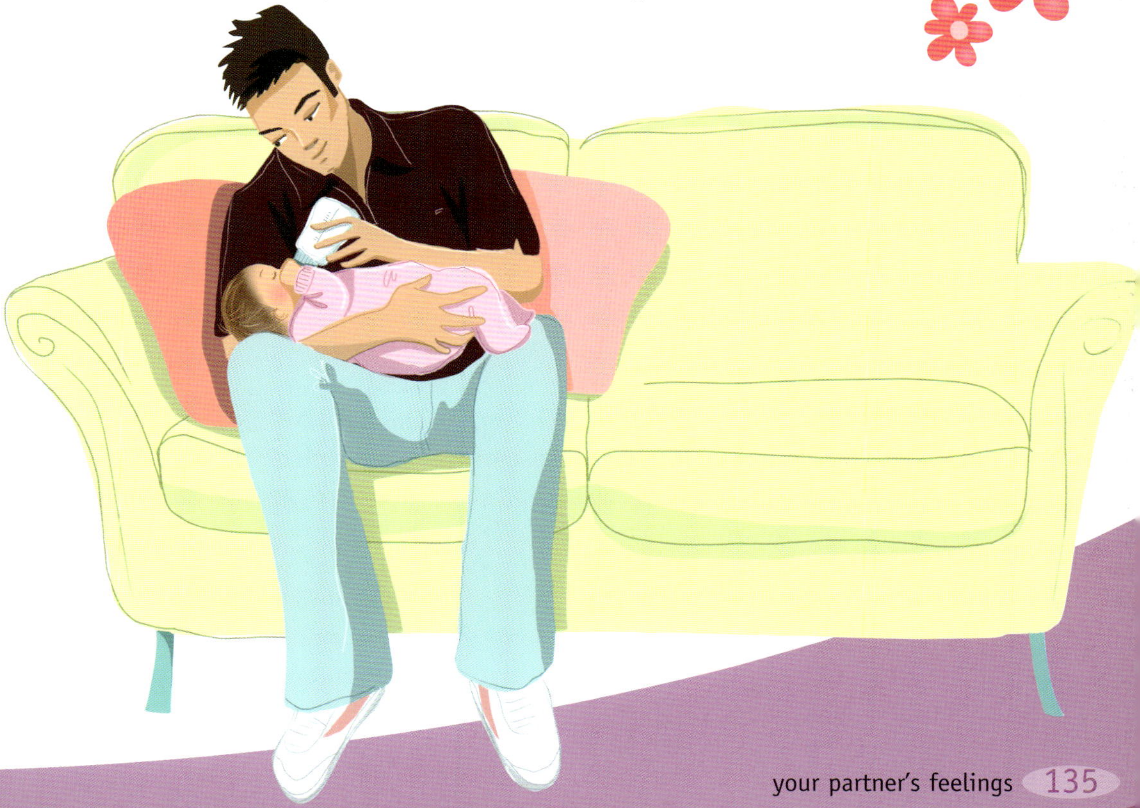

help!

getting help in the first few days

No matter how organized you were in preparing for the arrival of your baby, it is unlikely that you managed to account for everything. Perhaps you underestimated how tired you would feel post-delivery. Maybe you had to stay in the hospital longer than you planned. If you had a cesarean, you might be unable to cope physically during the first week or so at home. These are not failings on your part, it just takes time to adjust to a new life. Rather than add to your difficulties by trying to be a super-mom, take pride in accepting any offer of help you get for the first few days.

Your mom and mother-in-law are both likely to offer to stay during the first week. If you do not want them living with you, at least accept their help with daily chores. Take advantage of a friend who offers to baby-sit so you can take some time for yourself. Make the most of any aftercare you have from your midwife; have her help with difficulties breast-feeding, or with any concerns you have about the baby. Don't be afraid to ask for help.

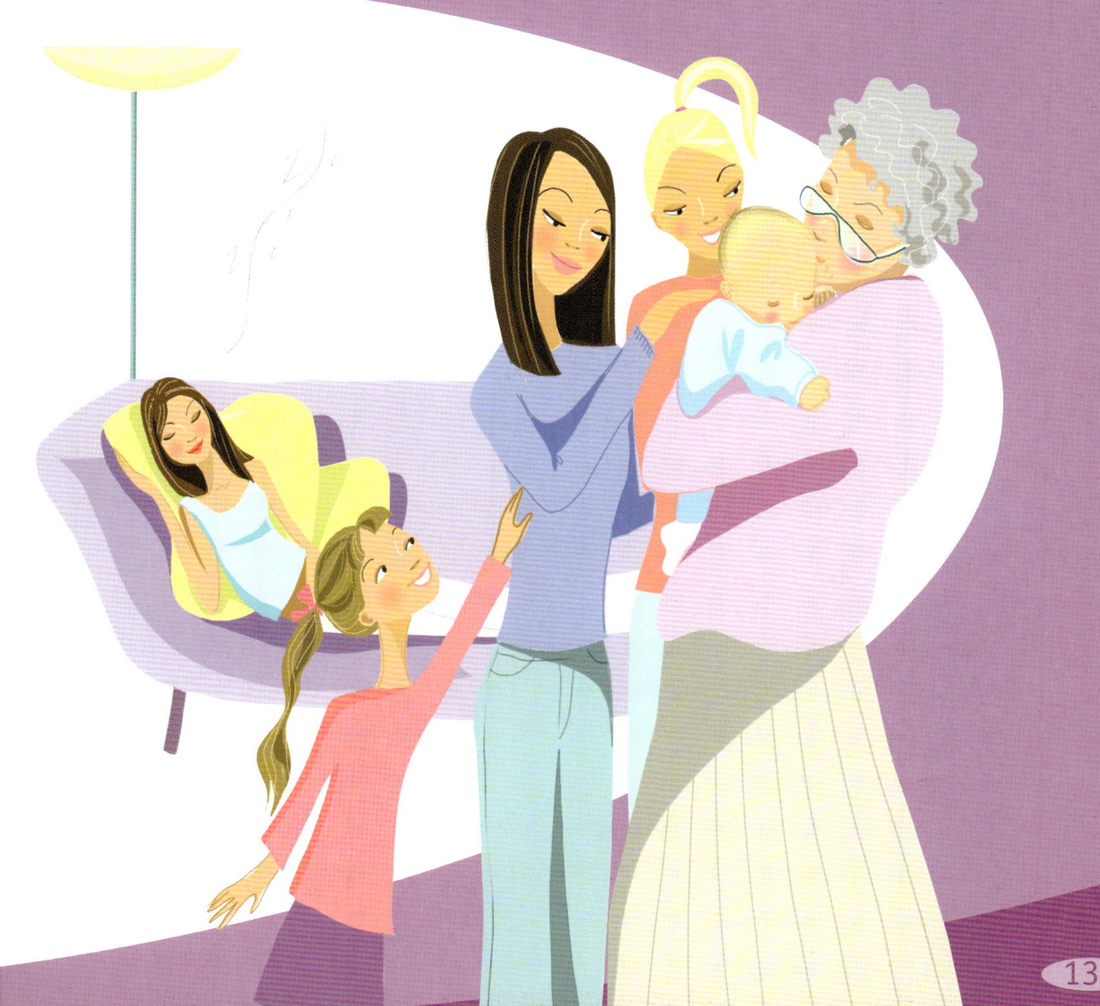

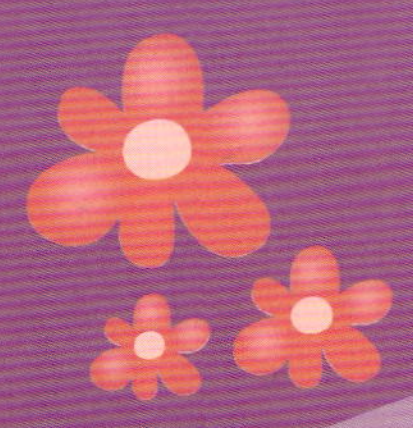

help!

choosing caregivers

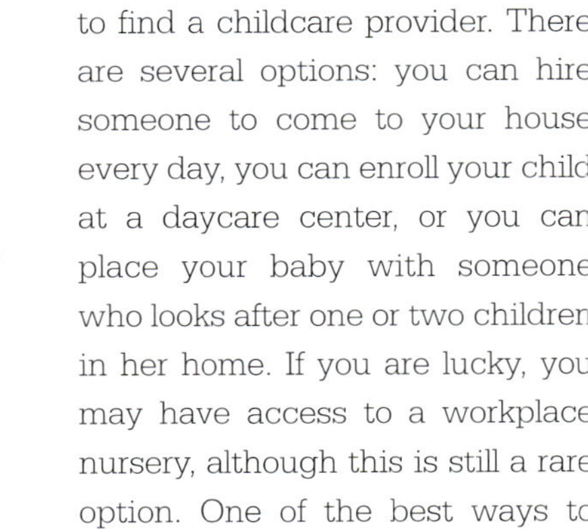

Unless one of you plans to stay home with the baby, you may have to find a childcare provider. There are several options: you can hire someone to come to your house every day, you can enroll your child at a daycare center, or you can place your baby with someone who looks after one or two children in her home. If you are lucky, you may have access to a workplace nursery, although this is still a rare option. One of the best ways to find a reliable caregiver is to ask your friends and neighbors.

There are a number of issues you should consider before confirming your choice. For example, will your caregiver:

- Give you daily communications about your child's day?
- Allow you to visit at any time without notice?
- Follow your guidelines regarding discipline or activities such as watching TV?
- Be trained in childcare and development and be properly licensed?
- Notify you well in advance of any changes in routine?

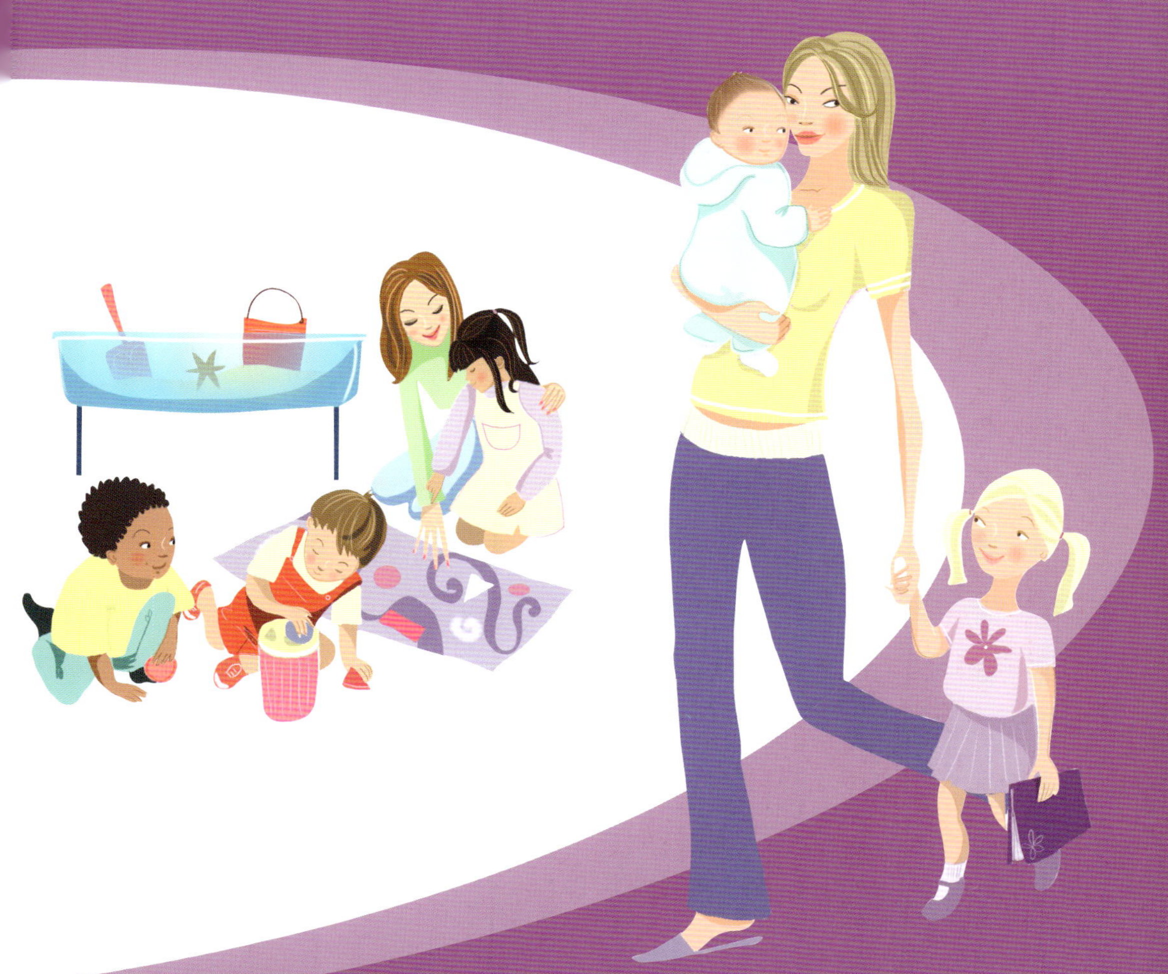

words, words, words, a glossary

amniotic fluid the cushioning fluid that surrounds the growing fetus from week four of the pregnancy.

breech position when the baby positions itself feet first at the onset of labor.

colostrum a yellowish substance produced by the breasts for the first three days after delivery, and that is full of vital nutrients for the baby, as well as antibodies to help it fight off infection.

edema a condition in late pregnancy when the legs and feet of the mother swell, owing to increased fluid levels in the body.

embryo the term used to describe the developing baby from week five through part of week 10, when the vital organs and major external features develop.

episiotomy an incision made in the perineum of the mother which may be made during labor in order to facilitate the birth.

fetus	the term used to describe the developing baby from the end of week 10 to birth, when all of the baby's systems mature.
hemorrhoids	swollen blood vessels that develop near or around the anus during the second trimester, as the uterus starts to put pressure on the veins.
lanugo	a fine hair that appears all over the growing fetus's body during the second trimester.
linea nigra	a dark line down the center of the abdomen of the mother that appears around the fourteenth week of pregnancy, and that is caused by an increased production of the pigment, melanin.
lochia	leftover blood and tissue discharged by the vagina in the days following delivery of the baby.
ovulation	the release of an egg from the ovary into the fallopian tube during the menstrual cycle.
oxytocin	the hormone that stimulates uterine contractions during labor, and that makes the mother's uterus contract after delivery.
placenta	the organ attached to the uterine wall, which facilitates the exchange of nutrients and waste between the mother and the growing fetus respectively.
prostaglandin	a hormone-like substance that stimulates muscle contractions, and that rises at the onset of labor.
quickening	the term used to describe the first, fluttery movements of the fetus.
vernix caseosa	a protective, white, cheese-like coating made from a mix of oil and skin cells, which appears during the second trimester and coats the skin of the fetus until birth.

index

First edition for North America published in 2004 exclusively by Ronnie Sellers Productions, Inc.

Conceived and created by Axis Publishing Limited
8c Accommodation Road, London NW11 8ED

Creative Director: Siân Keogh

Editorial Director: Anne Yelland

Art Director: Clare Reynolds

Managing Editor: Conor Kilgallon

Production: Jo Ryan

Illustrator: Lucy Truman

Published by Ronnie Sellers Productions, Inc.

P.O. Box 818, Portland, Maine 04104

(800) 625–3386 toll free

(207) 772–6814 fax

www.rsvp.com

rsp@rsvp.com

ISBN: 1–56906–549–7; LOC: 2004095076

Printed in Thailand

10 9 8 7 6 5 4 3 2 1

The author would like to thank Barbara Sutton Padovich, RNC, BSN, a nurse certified in inpatient obstetrics and fetal monitoring, for sharing her expertise and for reviewing the manuscript; and Dr. Sonya Naryshkin, MD, FIAC, for her many valuable comments and also for reviewing the manuscript.